What If Maslow Was Wrong?

Theresa A. Harvath • Mark Fedyk

What If Maslow Was Wrong?

Safety vs. Autonomy in Decision-Making for Older Adults

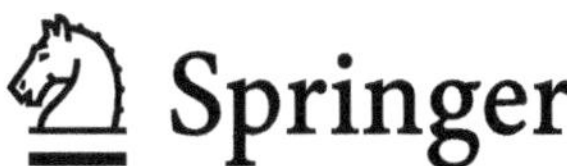

Springer

Theresa A. Harvath
School of Nursing, Retired
University of Minnesota
Minneapolis, MN, USA

Mark Fedyk
Bioethics Program, Division of General Internal Medicine and Bioethics
Department of Internal Medicine
School of Medicine
University of California, Davis
Sacramento, CA, USA

ISBN 978-3-032-14248-1 ISBN 978-3-032-14249-8 (eBook)
https://doi.org/10.1007/978-3-032-14249-8

This Springer imprint is published by the registered company Springer Nature Switzerland AG
The registered company address is: Gewerbestrasse 11, 6330 Cham, Switzerland

Preface: Safety and Impossible Choices

Many years ago, while walking on the Oregon beach, I encountered an older woman who would leave a lasting impression on my life and professional career. It was an early spring day, and the tide was out, leaving the beach open and clear except for the occasional driftwood log. As I walked, I could see an older woman in the distance walking toward me with two dogs in tow, one an energetic puppy that jumped and pawed at her, the other an older dog who waddled slowly by her side. She was a small woman wearing oversized rain boots and a long coat. She had a plaid scarf tied under her chin. Her sage green coat had a fur collar and was made of looped pile wool; the bottom 12 inches of the pile were brushed smooth from the dogs jumping up and pawing at her over the years.

As she made her way down the beach, she talked and played with the dogs. She stamped her foot at the young pup, sending him scurrying away after a treat she had thrown; then she slyly dropped a treat in front of the older dog, who was no match for the quickness of his younger rival. I sat on a driftwood log to watch the interactions between the woman and her two dogs, amused by her playfulness toward the one and moved by her tenderness toward the other.

I willed her to come and sit next to me and was delighted when she approached. We nodded a silent greeting. Then she said, "Its days like this at the beach when I would love to bring all the little blind children from Portland to come and play. I would station adults at the ocean's edge and just let the kiddos run and run without worry they would run into anything and get hurt." My heart, already touched by her interactions with her dogs, melted.

I asked her if she came to the beach often and she said she walked the same route every day, coming down one path from town, walking a stretch, and then heading back up another trail toward home. She told me that several years ago a winter storm had dropped a large piece of driftwood across the trail toward home and she had to climb over it to get past.

She then told me that just last week, she saw that someone had sawed the log in half and removed the center section that blocked her way. As she stood looking at the log a young man came up and asked her what she thought of his handiwork. She responded, "Are you the one who cut that log?" He said, smiling, "Yes, I could see you struggling to get over the log and didn't want you to fall." She replied, "You know what I'd like to do? I'd like to take that chainsaw, cut off your leg and beat you over the head with the bloody stump!" I was stunned (as I am sure the young man must have been) and nearly choked from laughter. I said, "What?" Not sure if I had heard her correctly. She repeated, "I told him I wanted to take that chainsaw, cut off his leg and beat him over the head with the bloody stump."

She went on to explain that while the log created an obstacle for her on the path, it had also provided a much-needed resting spot for her on her way home. The young man must have seen her struggle to get over the log but had not noticed that she rested there before continuing on her way.

Over the years, in the retelling of this story, I have come to understand (I think) the meaning of her dramatic response to his well-intentioned "good deed." The young man had assumed that he knew what the old woman needed and wanted, acting without checking with her first. It was an early lesson for me in my career in gerontological nursing that I could not presume to know what was best for the older adults in my care—I must ask them what they want and need.

This insight has been reinforced repeatedly in my interactions with older adults. Over the years, I have learned from many, many older patients that they believe I overestimate the risks involved in their choices (e.g., whether they are safe living at home). Or that although the risks may be real, the infringement on their quality of life, their autonomy, and their sense of control stemming from any attempts to mitigate the risks are also significant and must be factored into any decision. In other words, we must balance concerns for safety with concerns for quality of life and autonomy.

And yet, as simple as that concept seems on its face, it repeatedly challenges those of us involved in the care of older adults, including family caregivers who care for frail older family members and those with dementia. In situations where the expressed preferences of older adults involve some perceived risk (however remote), we tend to come down on the side of safety, ignoring, disregarding, or minimizing their stated preferences and the impact of caution on their quality of life. Instead, we advocate for strategies and interventions that promote safety (or, as we will explore further, the illusion of safety) believing that the good outweighs the impact on autonomy or quality of life. Now, don't get me wrong—I am not suggesting that we ignore serious threats to the safety of the older patients in our care. However, I have come to believe that we must not just protect their safety (to the extent possible), but also their autonomy and their quality of life. I believe that we need to do a better job of paying attention to their stated preferences regarding healthcare and living situations, that we need to understand what *they* believe is in their best interest, and that we need to ask, to listen and seek to accommodate those preferences that are integral to their quality of life. And I believe we should do this for older adults with dementia as well as those who remain cognitively intact.

I am a retired professor of gerontological nursing with over 40 years of experience with older adults and their family caregivers. I began my career as a nursing assistant in nursing homes while in nursing school. Over the course of my career, I have worked clinically with older adults in long-term care and acute care and with family caregivers in an outpatient clinic. As the geropsychiatric clinical nurse specialist at the Portland VA Nursing Skilled Care Unit, I consulted with staff and family members regarding older veterans with dementia, delirium, and/or depression. While at the Betty Irene Moore School of Nursing at the University of California Davis, I was the Principal Investigator and Founding Director of the Family Caregiving Institute. While in that role, I started an outpatient clinic for family caregivers for older adults. These experiences, along with those of countless students who were involved clinically with older adults, have enriched my career and strengthened my passion to improve the health and health care for frail older adults and their family caregivers. I have had the good fortune to learn with and from many colleagues who share my commitment to older adults. One of them is my co-author, Dr. Mark Fedyk.

Dr. Fedyk is a philosopher and ethicist in the School of Medicine at the University of California, Davis. He has a deep professional interest in decision-making about safety. Mark's work in the healthcare system has been different than mine. As an ethicist, he offers consultations to clinicians and researchers, which means that he usually does not work with patients directly. His role is to offer an ethical "second opinion" whenever doctors, nurses, and administrators get stuck making a difficult choice. Requests for an ethical "second opinion" often arise out of a desire for more—indeed, the most possible, usually—moral certainty. In this way, ethics consults are like the problems that caregivers face when making decisions for, or about, older adults in their lives. Everyone wants as much moral certainty as possible that they are "doing the right thing," but it is very difficult, if not impossible, to get there.

As you can imagine, safety comes up a lot in Mark's ethics consultations: no healthcare provider wants to do anything that would be unsafe for their patients. But it is also impossible for clinicians to provide care that comes with no risk whatsoever. We have never been able to identify a "perfectly safe, morally certain" solution to any ethical problem in the clinical arena. Because this tension—between safety and providing appropriate and meaningful medical care—is a fundamental part of making decisions about healthcare, it can be very hard to see clearly what exact course of action preserves "just the right amount" of safety, and in searching for that solution, it is usually the case that many possible choices arise that are attractive because they have the illusion of safety. Sometimes an ethics consult is effective simply because, like in the story above, we get clarity about what a patient really wants. It is often the case, however, that a dynamic tension exists between what the older adult prefers—based on their individual assessment of autonomy, quality of life, and risk—and the family's or healthcare provider's assessment of risk or their determination of what "should" be done.

This book is an attempt to combine our experiences and voices in a way that helps its readers figure out where to "put" safety when it comes to making decisions about the care of older adults. So, from here on, we'll start using "we" instead of "I," and of course, just like the woman in the story above, we do not advise ignoring safety altogether. The true difficulty comes in figuring out how to balance concerns for the older adult's safety and their preferences which reflect their desire for autonomy and quality of life.

Each chapter is organized, just like this one, around a real case that Terri or Mark encountered clinically. To protect people's identities, we've fictionalized elements of the cases, including the names of the patients and family members. But for each case, the central ethical dilemma is true to life, and the decisions and feelings we write about really did happen. Each chapter uses its case as inspiration to develop ideas about where to put safety alongside all the other things that usually must be considered when making decisions about the care of older adults.

Chapter 1 dives into the dilemma at the heart of many of the cases in this book: the idea, clearly exemplified in a popular (though perhaps inaccurate or overly simplified) interpretation of the work of the psychologist Abraham Maslow, that, when making difficult decisions, safety must be maximized before anything else in a person's life can have value. Chapter 2 looks at some of the different meanings the word "safety" has for clinicians and family caregivers. Having these different conceptual definitions out in the open helps avoid some all-too-common confusions about what kind of outcome we are looking for when we try to make things "safer" for an older adult.

Chapter 3 then turns to a more practical matter: if not maximizing safety, then how should people make difficult choices? We reflect on a case that provides an elegant example of how cost-benefit reasoning can be a way of balancing safety with other things that matter. We also bring into our discussion some of the most important concepts in the ethics of end-of-life care, the *best interest* versus *substituted judgment standards*, *advanced directives*, *daily-decision making*, and *durability of preferences*. Chapter 4 shifts perspective: starting from a brief description of an extremely common case, we survey some of the federal regulations and clinical literature that, because of their training and the influence of evidence-based care, most clinicians have in the back of their mind when they are working with older adults as they transition from living at home to living in a nursing home or some other kind of long-term care facility. This chapter works in tandem with Chap. 2 because it can facilitate more effective translation between patient and provider when talking about the difficult decisions that arise when these transitions occur. But it also introduces some high-level concepts and distinctions that we will explore more deeply in the remaining chapters.

Chapter 5 tackles one of the most clinically consequential of these high-level distinctions. It uses a case with extremely common features to pull apart the concepts of independence and autonomy and explain some of the ways in which you can use classical ethical principles to protect a person's autonomy even when they have diminished capacities. Chapter 6 then analyzes a case where attempts to "maximize safety" backfire. This chapter illustrates some of the pitfall and unintended consequences that can arise when people make decisions about the care of older adults that are sincerely intended to "put safety first." Chapter 7 examines a case that brings together nearly all the ethical ideas, both abstract and practical, that we introduce earlier in Chaps. 5 and 6. This chapter (we should tell you at the outset) is about a patient with dementia who masturbates before going to sleep. Because of how delicate and personal the case is, it helps us clarify some of the more complicated aspects of patient autonomy, as well as contrast ethical principlism with ethical pragmatism (see comments below for more on this).

Chapter 8 returns to some of the issues introduced in Chap. 4, but with a much more specific focus: it offers an explanation of some of the beliefs and principles—beyond a commitment to the Maslow-inspired idea that safety should be maximized—that can motivate providers to make decisions that seem to place all of the weight on safety. Chapter 9 is one half of this book's conclusion: we summarize the insights and lessons we are trying to share with you by offering you five "principles." However, we're aware that these principles won't help solve most cases—really, they function just to reduce the amount of stress and judgment families and caregivers may subject themselves to if they try to pursue moral certainty. Because of that, the second half of our conclusion comes in Chap. 10, where we share one of Terri's most wise ideas about what to do when you get to a point where no amount of scientific reasoning—and no logically coherent principles—help. Sadly, there probably is no way through life without getting into one of these situations.

How did a nurse and a philosopher end up co-writing a book? As we mentioned, Terri and Mark worked together to provide consultations for patients and caregivers who were burdened with *impossible choices* about caregiving. This book emerges out of the conversations—sometimes lasting hours!—that followed each of these consultations. These consultations illustrated an important truth: that there was no silver bullet in trying to figure out how much weight to give to considerations of safety. There is no algorithm or principle or formula that could be used to help caregivers of patients with dementia figure out the optimum balance of safety versus quality of life. You cannot reduce decisions about care to filling out a checklist or following some set of highly standardized best practices. Indeed, we observed that the very opposite was normal. For caregivers of persons with dementia, often the best that we could offer was the recognition—and *validation*—that they were being forced to make a series of impossible choices.

What is an impossible choice? It is a choice where there is both no obvious "right" or "correct" answer that all involved can agree on, no certainty about what to do or what the consequences will be, but a decision cannot be avoided. Just kicking the can down the road is not a solution. Another word for an impossible choice is a choice that is "forced" by life upon the people who must make it: a family caregiver, a brother and a sister, or a single daughter cannot avoid having their life interrupted—perhaps even completely taken over—by attempting to figure out what to do about something that does not have a perfectly rational, perfectly scientific, perfectly obvious solution. Validating that a choice really is an *impossible choice* means that it is OK—normal—to feel overwhelmed, defeated, or demoralized in the face of such a choice. It is normal to feel ill-prepared to make such an important decision or that there *should* be a single right decision—but then realizing that there isn't. That really is facing the reality of the situation.

It shouldn't be a surprise for us to share with you that we—Terri and Mark—don't agree about everything. In fact, our training in ethics explains the biggest area where we have different beliefs and values. Terri, being trained as a clinician, has been socialized to see ethical dilemmas —whether they generate impossible choices—as opportunities to apply an ethical framework called *principlism*. This framework is easy to learn because it says that all ethical problems in healthcare can be solved by applying one of four principles: autonomy, justice, beneficence, and non-maleficence. Figuring out what to do when you face a dilemma, then, is figuring out which of the principles to apply, and the best order to apply the principles. For instance, in a case where a patient is refusing a life-saving blood transfusion in an emergency situation, do we place autonomy (which usually means letting patients determine the course of their care, even if their choices aren't what other people would choose in the same circumstances) ahead of non-maleficence (which usually means ensuring that patients aren't harmed by the course of their care)? And do we even care about justice (which usually means that scarce healthcare resources be used in an equitable fashion) and beneficence (which usually means that a patient should benefit in some way from any medical or clinical interventions)? For Terri, many of the dilemmas involving care of older adults involve failures to "rank" autonomy high enough. As we will explore in the later chapters, considerations of safety are very easily tied to the logic of beneficence or non-maleficence in a way that costs patients their autonomy when safety (i.e., beneficence or non-maleficence) is ranked higher than autonomy. Terri disagrees with the view that safety is *always* the *most* important concept when making decisions about care for older adults—and so she also disagrees with the view that beneficence and non-maleficence should almost always be the two principles which rank highest when deciding what to do in a case.

Mark agrees with Terri about the principles of beneficence and non-maleficence: rarely should they be ranked higher than autonomy. But he disagrees with Terri that the first thing to do when facing an ethical dilemma is to figure out which principles should be ranked highest when trying to figure out what to do. This attitude is, like Terri's default attitude, also a by-product of his training. Coming from a background in academic ethics, his first reaction to a case is not to ask which of the four principles is most applicable to the case—but instead: Which unique ethical framework is most applicable to the case? It could be principlism, of course, but it could also be any number of alternatives. Utilitarianism, care ethics, or ethical pragmatism (Mark's favorite) might be the best "cognitive tool" to use to think through the case at hand.

What we found interesting is that, while Mark and Terri's training in ethics was very different, they share what tends to be a nonconventional view of how ethics should inform clinical practice. Terri arrived there through an inductive process built from clinical situations where the principlism approach was awkward at best, Mark through a more deductive, theory-driven process. They agree that pragmatism usually offers a much more compassionate and humane approach for dealing with an impossible choice than principlism. However, ethical pragmatism requires more patience and a greater tolerance for uncertainty than principlism when it is applied in real-world settings.

For most of this book, this difference between Mark and Terri will not matter. Our shared thesis is that safety does not always matter the most when facing impossible choices in the care of older adults. However, we have dedicated a meaningful portion of Chap. 7 to exhibiting the difference between one of the most popular versions of principlism—specifically, a Kantian approach to thinking about autonomy—and ethical pragmatism, as the case that this chapter is about is almost perfectly designed to provide a useful contrast between these two ethical frameworks.

This book is written primarily for anyone facing an impossible choice when caring for an older adult. It is also written for students in health professions schools who will find themselves sooner or later working closely with caregivers (both family and paid) who are facing impossible choices. (For the students, we've included discussion questions at the end of each chapter.) Each of the chapters is about a different aspect of the tensions that arise when our efforts to keep frail, older adults safe diminishes their quality of life, quashes their autonomy, or thwarts their expressed preferences. As we've said, the overriding theme of this book is that either maximizing or strongly prioritizing safety is not an effective way of dealing with most impossible choices involved in the care of older adults. But throughout, and even though we'll offer plenty of suggestions, our aim will not be to tell our readers what to do. Instead, we hope this book will help you feel less alone and overwhelmed by the presence of an impossible choice in your life. We hope it gives you ways of thinking about these decisions to uncover the real risks to safety (and not just the imagined ones) and the older adults' preferences regarding autonomy and quality of life.

Minneapolis, MN, USA Theresa A. Harvath

Sacramento, CA, USA Mark Fedyk

Contents

What If Maslow Was Wrong? 1

1.1 Case Illustration

Thomas Kane was a 79-year-old man with moderate dementia who was admitted to the veteran nursing home for rehabilitation following surgical repair of a hip fracture. Shortly after his admission, he was diagnosed with aspiration pneumonia. After a thorough evaluation, it was determined that he had a swallowing disorder that was likely related to an intraoperative stroke. Mr. Kane was found to be a "silent" aspirator, meaning he tended to aspirate food into his lungs without any discernable coughing or choking.

Mr. Kane was assigned to the Progressive Self-Feeding Program to retrain his swallowing abilities. Unfortunately, his dementia inhibited his ability to relearn how to swallow safely. He underwent mental status testing, and the psychologist found that he lacked decisional capacity and was unable to accurately appreciate his risk for aspiration. Consequently, the speech pathologist, occupational therapist, and dietician recommended that he be placed on a pureed diet with thickened liquids.

Mr. Kane hated his pureed diet. He was convinced that the pureed pancake he was served was actually raw pancake batter. He complained about taking a spoonful of something red, thinking it was strawberries, only to realize it was beets. He would say in a wistful voice, "I just can't imagine life without another bite of Marie Callendar's boysenberry pie!"

Despite being on a pureed diet, Mr. Kane continued to experience repeated episodes of aspiration pneumonia. Therefore, a G-tube was placed, and orders were written for him to be NPO (which means "nil per os," which is Latin for "nothing by mouth"). However, Mr. Kane always had spare change in his pocket and would freely avail himself of the vending machines, forgetting that he was not supposed to eat anything orally. His choices included cookies, candies, and snacks that had peanuts and other crunchy textures. He continued to develop aspiration pneumonia, and it was presumed that either he could not handle his own secretions or he was aspirating foods that he acquired from the vending machines.

T. A. Harvath, M. Fedyk, *What If Maslow Was Wrong?*,
https://doi.org/10.1007/978-3-032-14249-8_1

During an interdisciplinary team meeting, the staff debated what to do to try to address Mr. Kane's bouts of aspiration pneumonia. Some staff argued that, based on concerns for quality of life, Mr. Kane should be allowed to eat a full texture diet, despite the risks involved. Others asserted that because Mr. Kane lacked decisional capacity, he could not consent to the risks involved, and therefore additional efforts should be made to limit his access to food. Mr. Kane's niece (his only living relative) was consulted about the decision. She stated, "Oh please don't make me decide what to do. I don't want to be responsible for either ending his life or ruining his quality of life."

1.2 Clinical Dilemma and Maslow's Hierarchy of Needs

Mr. Kane's situation is a classic example of a common dilemma encountered by staff who are trying to implement care that prioritizes the preferences and values of the patient—a practice that is complicated whenever a patient has dementia or when a patient has preferences or values that entail some degree of clinical risk. These situations often pit concerns for safety against the older person's autonomy, expressed preferences, quality of life, or other things of value that cannot be reduced to safety. Time and again, when faced with this dilemma, we tend to come down on the side of safety, often citing Maslow's hierarchy of needs (Maslow 1943) as justification for prioritizing safety. Because Mr. Kane's dysphagia could be life-threatening—or at least a situation in which there are clear and obvious medical risks that, if not managed properly, could lead to profoundly negative outcomes for Mr. Kane—assuring his safety seems paramount. Indeed, as Maslow himself noted (and we'll quote him below), we tend to forget about a person's higher needs and values when we believe that the person is facing an immediate threat to safety.

What is Maslow's hierarchy of needs? Interestingly, Maslow did not provide a list of all of the levels of his hierarchy, nor did he provide a complete list of the needs at each of those levels. So, to present his hierarchy as it is frequently used in healthcare decision-making, some amount of interpretation is called for. With that clarification, here is a common representation of the needs in Maslow's hierarchy:

The hierarchy is often depicted as a pyramid (Fig. 1.1) where the most fundamental needs are at the base and other needs placed in a hierarchy of importance, ending with self-actualization at the top.

But before diving into Maslow's hierarchy, we need to say something important about the concept *of* a hierarchy and, more specifically, the concept of a dependency hierarchy (which is how Maslow's hierarchy is commonly interpreted in healthcare). A dependency hierarchy is a collection of things that are organized according to the following rule: you cannot have any of the things in the upper levels unless you've already got the stuff at the bottom. So, a common interpretations of Maslow's hierarchy is this: as you go up the hierarchy, you must satisfy *all* in the lower-level needs to even attempt to satisfy *any* of the needs at a higher level. Since safety is one

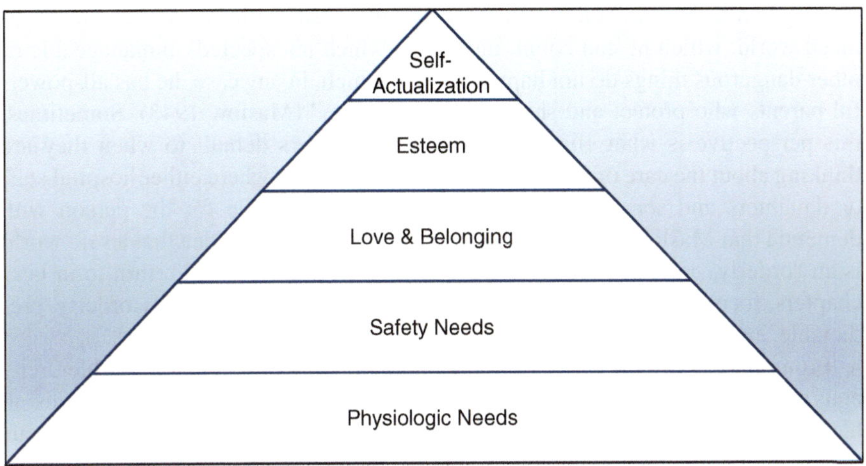

Fig. 1.1 Common depiction of Maslow's hierarchy of needs

of the two bottom levels of Maslow's hierarchy, this implies that unless you have safety then you cannot have anything of the higher levels—no love, no esteem, and no self-actualization without safety.

Psychologists in the early twentieth century often thought about human growth and development using dependency hierarchies or, as they also called them, stages (e.g., Erickson's stages of development). In practice, this often meant that they put forward scientific theories that held that most people tend to live their lives passing through each level or stage: first, you get the level 1 resources, then you use those to get the level 2 resources, and so on. Then, at the end of life, you might go through some of all the stages in reverse order: if you've reached stage 4, dementia might shift you back to stage 3, then eventually stage 2, and then finally to level 1.

1.3 In Maslow's Own Words

Let us now turn to some of Maslow's own observations about his hierarchy. Here is what Maslow had to say about needs at different levels. "If all the needs [of the lowest level, i.e. the physiological needs] are unsatisfied, and the [person] is then dominated by the physiological needs, all other needs may become simply non-existent or be pushed into the background" (Maslow 1943). As we explained above, this implies that a person cannot pursue any of the higher resources if their most basic, physiological needs are not met. The same is true of the next level, a person's "safety" needs, the essence of which is freedom from danger. Maslow uses the perspective of a child to explain the emergence of this level of need: the "average child in our society generally prefers a safe, orderly, predictable, organized world, which he can count, on, and in which unexpected, unmanageable or other dangerous things do not happen, and in which, in any case, he has all-powerful parents who protect and shield him from harm" (Maslow 1943). Sometimes, this perspective is what clinicians or family members default to when they are thinking about the care of persons with dementia, except where either hospital staff or daughters and sons, nieces, and nephews play the role for the person with dementia that Maslow thinks parents play for the child. (The idea that a safe world is an "orderly, predictable, organized" world is one that we will return to in later chapters, focusing on the idea that clinical spaces must be extremely orderly, predictable, and organized.)

From these remarks, it is easy to see how the idea of a dependency hierarchy emerges. When a person's physiological needs are met, it allows them to focus on having their safety needs met; when the safety needs are met, it allows them to focus on having their love and belonging needs met; and so on up the hierarchy.

But notice that this way of thinking about how the needs are organized does not yet tell us whether we should try to maximize all the individual needs as we go up the levels or whether our job is to try to find a way of balancing the different needs. Does safety need to be at "10" before a person can find love? Or is 8 enough? It seems plausible that balancing is the most realistic way to think about Maslow's hierarchy: a collection of "5"s, "6"s, "7"s, and"8"s might be the most stable way of satisfying all of the needs in the hierarchy.

These questions help us see an important property of dependency hierarchies: the relation of dependency that holds between the levels and the stages is more complex than a simple linear progression. Thus, prioritizing safety by insisting that it be no less than "10" over quality of life in cases like Mr. Kane's because Maslow's hierarchy says safety is more important than other human needs may help us to justify that decision, but it doesn't mean we have made the "right" decision from either the ethical or the psychological perspecitves.

If we look at accepted practices in long-term care related to managing risk, we can begin to uncover the complexity involved in making these kinds of decisions. If, for example, Mr. Kane were determined to have decisional capacity, the staff would likely have honored his desire to maximize his quality of life and not tried to prevent him from taking food orally. This suggests that having the freedom to choose supersedes restrictions related to concerns for safety (not in all cases, see Chap. 6 for more on this topic). So, this is one reason why "maximizing safety above all else" is not necessarily congruent with Maslow's scientific thoughts.

Admittedly, balancing *all* of one's needs at each of the levels of the hierarchy is much harder to put into practice than maximizing one or two of needs located at the lower levels of Maslow's hierarchy. You can see the difference between maximizing and balancing clearly in Mr. Kane's niece's response to his frequent bouts of aspiration pneumonia: "Oh please don't make me decide what to do. I don't want to be responsible for either ending his life or ruining his quality of life." Her statement reflects the difficulty of balancing safety with quality of life, because she recognizes that, for Mr. Kane, it simply isn't possible to maximize just one or the other. Balancing all a person's needs is hard! Yet, that is the work that clinicians and family caregivers often find themselves facing.

1.4 Hierarchies and Balancing Versus Maximizing

It is important to note that Maslow did not actually draw a diagram representing his dependency hierarchy in his famous 1943 article. Subsequent authors and researchers—for example, Eliopoulos (2014), Mauk (2014), and Touhy and Jett (2014)—have tended to portray his ideas in diagrams shaped like pyramids, just as we did above (Fig. 1.1). This practice reinforces the assumption we have just been discussing, that it is usually that the lower levels aren't just necessary, but each of the needs at all of the lower levels *must* be maximized, in order to secure the higher levels.

We want to suggest that part of the motivation here may be less a concern to describe human nature deeply and more a matter of conceptual convenience. Why? If you look at all the needs listed in Table 1.1, there are at least 20 distinct needs that are to be satisfied. Notice how much more complex it is to try to find a way to balance all 20 needs versus just trying to maximize the needs individually. The former involves a process of never-ending tweaking, measuring, and adjusting, always paying attention to how putting time and energy into meeting needs for achievement or bodily security impact needs like moral safety or the need for restful sleep. A clinical team who takes over the work of *balancing* all a person's needs versus maximizing a few lower-level individual needs just has a lot more work to do.

We can explain a further reason that the distinction between maximizing individual needs and balancing all a person's needs matters. When clinicians and family members talk about a patient's quality of life, they almost always have some kind of

Table 1.1 Maslow's hierarchy of needs

Need	Definition
Self-actualization	The freedom to choose the form and course of one's being and the understanding of the nature of one's being to be able to make choices about form and course that are congruent with one's nature
Esteem	Self-respect, self-esteem, the respect and esteem of others, good reputation, opportunities to make meaningful contributions to the world
The love needs	Giving and receiving love, giving and receiving affection, social belonging, friendship, partnership in marriage
The safety needs	Freedom from threat of injury, of illness, of pain, routine and social order, good parenting, freedom from criminal activity, freedom from illnesses that disturb cognitive function
The basic or physiological needs	Homeostasis, sleep, sex, physical connection, excretion

process for keeping the various needs to be balanced in mind—they are never suggesting maximizing *only* quality of life. So, a plan for a patient's *quality of life* is some plan for balancing what can be balanced within the patient's specific situation, given what is going on at all levels in the hierarchy.

It is worth noting that the notion of the pyramid is not wrong per se; rather, it is when we use it as an oversimplified approach that can justify clinical priorities and decisions we go awry. Unfortunately, in our experience, the idea that safety should be maximized at all costs (because that is what Maslow's hierarchy appears to show) usually leads clinicians to ignore the various ways in which "higher" needs are still real and achievable for a patient. Despite his dementia and impairments to his upper GI function, Mr. Kane is still able to problem solve, pursue activities that reflect his self-conception, and articulate very clearly the essential role that Marie Callendar's boysenberry pie played in his quality of life. Just because we can't assure an individual's safety doesn't mean the needs at higher levels cannot be achieved. If we used the pyramid in our clinical decision-making, it should be to inform us that, with safety compromised, we might need to explore other avenues to achieve higher needs than through the impossible restoration of absolute safety. Because of this, the scope of what gets balanced and how probably must change: some compromises around how much and how often Mr. Kane eats pie are probably inevitable.

1.5 Biological Versus Logical Needs

Maslow appeared to struggle to say clearly what the relationship between the levels in his hierarchy is. In another article, he wrote that the basic needs are arranged "in a hierarchy of less

or greater priority or potency" and that when the lower needs are unmet they "dominate" the higher needs until they are fulfilled (Maslow 1954, 59). Maslow seems to have in mind that conscious motivation organizes around having unfulfilled needs fulfilled, but that is almost a definition of what a need is, rather than an explanation of how they can be organized in a hierarchy.

At this point, we want to offer a distinction that helps us say much more explicitly what the relationship is, beyond that of dependency, between the levels in Maslow's hierarchy. One interpretation of Maslow's hierarchy is to interpret it as a *logical* hierarchy. This tries to further refine what the conditional "if the lower needs are not satisfied, then the higher needs cannot be satisfied either" means in our discussion of dependency hierarchies from above. What makes a dependency hierarchy a logical hierarchy is if it adds the following condition: a hierarchy of needs is a logical hierarchy if it is impossible for the higher needs to be satisfied unless the lower needs are *maximally* satisfied. This is a very strong claim, because it means that the most basic needs—physiological needs and safety needs—must have absolute priority over all other needs that a person might have.

The alternative to a logical hierarchy of needs is a *biological* hierarchy of needs, an idea which, thankfully, can be illustrated. Here then is a drawing that Dr. Katarzyna Malin, a veterinarian and scientific illustrator at UC Davis, made for us.

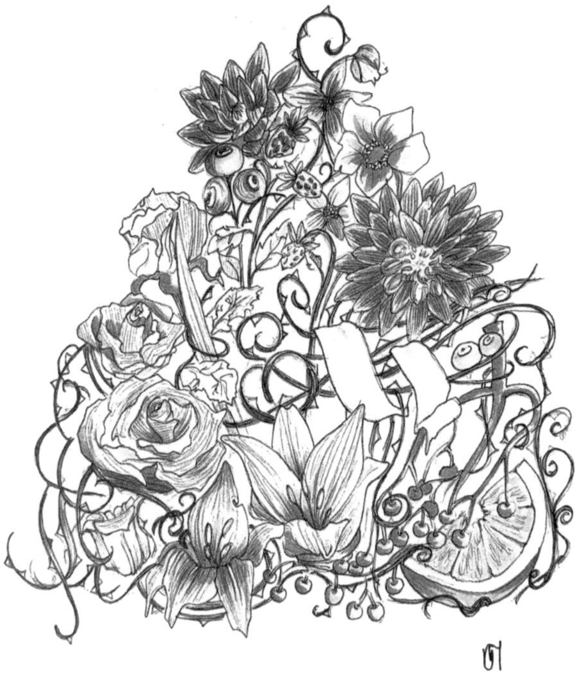

What this picture shows is an entangled biological system of flowers, fruits, stems, berries, and leaves, all in their own unique way balanced together. If you squint, you can see five levels in the picture, and in some important sense, the upper parts of the tangle are supported by the lower parts—but the whole system has found a way of growing together. Because of this, this drawing captures the idea of needs being balanced. But the drawing also captures two important further points: First, if a stem or a flower in the lower part of the tangle were to wither and die or some of the berries to be eaten, the tangle itself could adapt to the change; the whole organic system would not collapse if a flower were removed. Second, there is no sense in which you can talk about the dahlias or the roses or the berries in the illustration as being "maximized": they simply are the size that they are, figuring in as coherent part in an organic whole.

The alternative to a logical hierarchy of needs, then, is a biological hierarchy of needs. Biological hierarchies are tangled, but adaptable, systems that, literally, are living systems and remain living partly because each of the "needs" is balanced with all the other needs.

So, rather, than thinking about Mr. Kane's needs as factors or qualities that should be maximized, we can reimagine Mr. Kane's needs as a biological hierarchy, like so:

1. Boysenberry Pie
2. Preservation of Dignity
3. Effective Caregiving
4. Stable and Consistent Healthcare
5. Breating, Food, Water, Sleep,
Excreation, Homeostasis
1.
2.
3.
4.
5.

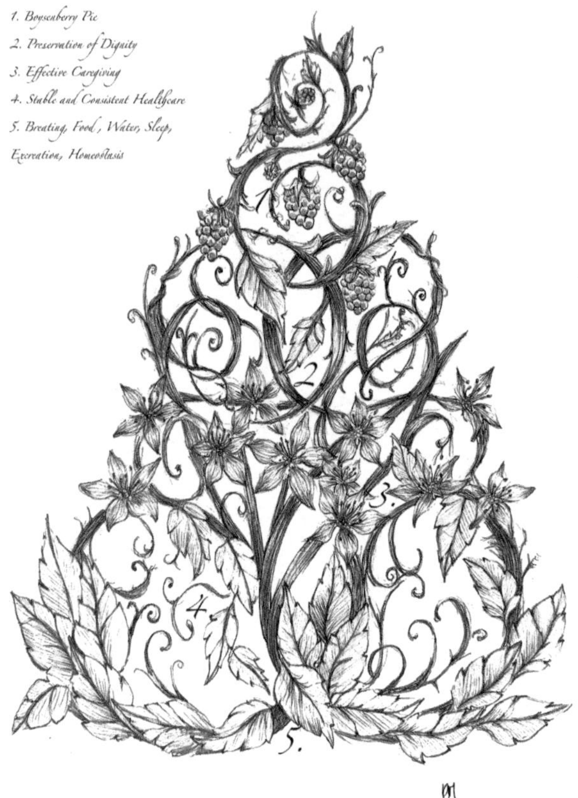

This is a less lively, less dense biological hierarchy than the first illustration above—a concession to the reality of Mr. Kane's reduced capacities. Nevertheless, it does capture something important about Mr. Kane: his life is still a life in which his "highest" needs can be satisfied by creatively finding ways to balance their satisfaction with the satisfaction of his more basic needs. At the top of this picture are boysenberries, ripe for the picking.

Now, we aren't suggesting that every patient needs to hire a scientific illustrator to have their own hierarchy of needs depicted. Rather, we offer these two illustrations as a way of priming your imagination: if we can imagine unique biological hierarchies of needs for each patient, this dramatically clarifies how to ensure the patient's quality of life does not get ignored when planning a course of care. In Mr. Kane's case, the picture above could have rather vividly helped them understand the importance of boysenberry pie—and this understanding is not in any way trivial. Anything that helps the people caring for Mr. Kane become more coordinated with each other is a step in the right direction. So, we encourage you to think about everyone as having integrated and entangled needs that must be constantly brought into balance with one another—that needs should be thought of as forming a biological hierarchy—i.e., a tangled but living system that forms a unique organic whole.

1.6 Drawing Your Own Hierarchy of Needs

Indeed, we also want to suggest that it may be helpful to try sketching an individualized pyramid of needs for any patient or family member for whom you are caring. This may help you see the unique arrangement of needs that characterize that person's life. Here, we can suggest two simple rules for drawing these customized pyramids of needs: The first is that pyramids that are "tall and skinny" (like Mr. Kane's) will usually be better, all things being equal, than pyramids that are "short and flat." "Tall and skinny" means that the customized pyramid has only as many layers needed to reflect salient issues, concerns, and patient preferences, even if it means that the total number of needs that are being actively balanced is fewer than an alternative customized pyramid that focuses on the largest possible number of most basic needs. "Tall and skinny" also suggests that the needs at different levels are not necessarily more important than needs at other levels. So, while ease of breathing is important for Mr. Kane, it is important that it not completely override his need for dignity and respect. In contrast, "short and flat" pyramids (like the ones often used to depict Maslow's hierarchy) suggest that needs at a lower level (the wider level) are much more important than the needs at the top which take up less area of the overall pyramid.

The second rule is that "the balance is always imperfect, and it will constantly be changing." This rule is a helpful reminder that, when trying to balance needs at different levels of a dependency hierarchy, rather than focusing primarily a select few of basic needs, the complexity of the work means we need to have modest expectations about how successful we will be and even more modest expectations about the long-term stability any "good enough" balancing of needs we happen to achieve. Notice that Mr. Kane's pyramid isn't perfectly symmetrical and that some stalks are thicker than others. And while the roots are essential, so are the leaves and the flowers.

1.7 Back to the Case

Now, you may be wondering what happened to Mr. Kane. Through intensive (and repeated) interdisciplinary discussions, it was finally concluded that, despite our best efforts, we (his care team) were not able to prevent Mr. Kane from developing aspiration pneumonia. Even with the closest supervision possible during meals, his doctors and nurses were not able to determine when he aspirated foods. In addition, we felt uncomfortable restricting his access to the vending machines because it made him feel as though he was disobeying orders, resulting in profuse apologies. The team also had to acknowledge that even when he was NPO he developed aspiration pneumonia.

Eventually, the chaplain asked the question: "Would we think about this differently if we saw Mr. Kane as terminally ill?" What a great question! It immediately changed how we thought about his situation and the options that were available to us. We decided that even though we could not prevent his aspiration pneumonia, what we could do was try to respect his quality of life, for whatever time he had left to live, by giving him access to the foods that provided him pleasure. His care team also changed his orders to reflect comfort care measures only, that he should be DNR (do not resuscitate), and that we would not hospitalize him for pneumonia (he hated going to the hospital). He was eventually discharged to an assisted living facility where he was permitted a full-texture diet. He died about 6 months later from an apparent, though unwitnessed, aspiration.

1.8 Challenges We Encountered

It seems that Mr. Kane lived the rest of his life with his various needs balanced with one another. True, there is a chance that he could live slightly longer if he had remained on NPO or had been rushed to the hospital when his pneumonia returned, but this would have meant that he lived without some of his higher needs going satisfied. The pyramid for his life would have lost some of its higher levels—it would have been too short and flat.

There are a host of additional challenges that came up as we waded through this challenging and complex case:

- *What will his family think?* As noted, we tried to defer this tough decision to Mr. Kane's niece. She immediately recognized the undesirable possibilities and summed them up stating that she didn't want to be the person responsible for "either ending his life or ruining his quality of life." Still, we kept the conversation with her open, discussing our concerns, helping her see our struggle with this dilemma. In so doing, she was able to understand that we were trying to do the best thing we could for her uncle, taking his stated preferences into account.
- *If he chokes when I feed him, will I be responsible for his death?* It is essential that we did not ignore the real concerns expressed by staff who worked with Mr. Kane daily. They were very fond of him and wanted to protect him from any harm. Again, we talked through our concerns as a team and reaffirmed our person-centered values that were reflected in other aspects of the care we provided (e.g., a cafeteria line where the residents could freely make food selections no matter what their diagnoses). We also discussed the importance of quality of life, even at the cost of quantity of life, a message that our residents spoke of at weekly community meetings. We would, of course, respond to a choking episode knowing how distressing that is for the person choking and those witnessing the choking. We believed that was consistent with our commitment to keeping him comfortable.
- *What would the newspapers say if they got a hold of this?* This is an interesting argument that can carry a lot of weight but, in reality, seems rather remote. Still, we talked about how we might defend our decision should the need arise. We concluded that this was a clear dilemma without a singular right answer (if there were one, it would be obvious to us all). We also concluded that if others heard the whole story they might be as compelled as we were and at least acknowledge our decision

had validity, even if they did not completely agree. So, we documented our decision carefully. We documented that we understood there were risks involved in supporting Mr. Kane's expressed preferences, but that there were also risks involved in thwarting them, risks to his quality of life and his sense of control. We documented the rationale for our decision as clearly as we could.

It is impossible to know whether we made the right decision for Mr. Kane. Learning that he had died of an apparent aspiration or choking event (it was not witnessed) gave us pause and reminded us of the gravity of the decisions we were making on behalf of residents with diminished decisional capacity. Interestingly, there is a growing body of research to suggest that enteral feeding for persons with dementia do not promote and may, in fact, reduce survival rates (Cintra et al. 2014; Alvarez-Fernandez et al. 2005; Candy et al. 2009). So, while many health professionals believe that feeding tubes are safer than oral feeding in older adults with dementia who have dysphagia, they may increase the risk for aspiration pneumonia and death by reducing the pressure gradient between the stomach and the esophagus. An important part of evidence-based practice is recognizing that we can't be sure whether a particular patient will benefit from the evidence-based intervention or be in the group that doesn't.

Again, we'll never know whether we made the right choices for Mr. Kane. But we believe we made the best decision possible, given what we knew at the time. We also believe that the time and effort we took to deliberate the decision was what, at a minimum, we owed Mr. Kane. In the following chapters, we will dig into additional strategies and principles that we hope are useful for dealing with these kinds of complex challenges.

Discussion and Reflection Questions

1. The staff at the nursing home were concerned that Mr. Kane was helping himself to hard-textured foods from the vending machines. What strategies might the staff consider for reducing the likelihood that he would ingest foods that were not pureed? What are the advantages and limitations to these different strategies? What impact might these interventions have on Mr. Kane's quality of life?
2. If you learned that Mr. Kane was terminally ill and likely had only 6 more months to live, how would this information impact your opinion of what should be done regarding his diet?
3. What would your customized pyramid of needs include? How might this change over time?

References

Alvarez-Fernandez B, Garcia-Ordonez MA, Martinez-Manzanares C, Gomez-Huelgas R (2005) Survival of a cohort of elderly patients with advanced dementia: nasogastric tube feeding as a risk factor for mortality. Int J Geriatr Psychiatry 20(4):363–370

Candy B, Sampson EL, Jones L (2009) Enteral tube feeding in older people with advanced dementia: a Cochrane systematic review. Int J Palliat Nurs 15(8):396–404

Cintra MT, de Rezenda NA, de Moraes EN, Cunha LC, da Gama Torres HO (2014) A comparison of survival, pneumonia and hospitalization in patients with advanced dementia and dysphagia receiving either oral or enteral nutrition. J Nutr Health Aging 18(10):894–899

Eliopoulos C (2014) Gerontological Nursing, 8th edn. Lippincott, Williams & Wilkins, Philadelphia

Maslow AH (1943) A theory of human motivation. Psychol Rev 50(4):370–396

Maslow AH (1954) The role of basic need gratification in psychological theory. In: Maslow AH (ed) Motivation and personality. Harper & Row Publishers, Inc, New York

Mauk KL (2014) Gerontological nursing: competencies for care. Jones & Bartlett, Burlington

Touhy TA, Jett KF (2014) Ebersole and Hess' gerontological nursing and healthy aging, 4th edn. Mosby, St. Louis

2 Different Meanings of "Safety"

2.1 Case Illustration

Madge Isaacson was a 101-year-old woman with moderate dementia who lived by herself in her tiny, two-story home. While the house was gradually falling into disrepair, she enjoyed tinkering in the basement, going through her old photos, and puttering in the kitchen. Over the years, she had adopted stray animals from the neighborhood—an injured rabbit, an abandoned kitten. However, for the past 5–6 years, she had started to feed the feral cats in the neighborhood, allowing them to come into her house on cold, rainy nights. Although this resulted in unsanitary conditions in her home, she seemed to enjoy the cats and took great pleasure in their company.

*Mrs. Isaacson had a son and daughter who lived nearby and provided as much assistance as she would allow, which wasn't much. They had tried repeatedly to remove the cats, much to Mrs. Isaacson's displeasure. They had also tried to introduce some additional services (*e.g.*, home-delivered meals, housekeeping services, and a daily companion), but Mrs. Isaacson quickly dispensed with them all, asserting that they were a waste of money and insisting she was fine on her own.*

Over time, Mrs. Isaacson grew weaker and weaker. She ate irregularly and started to lose weight. She fell down the basement steps one evening, sustaining a 2-inch laceration on the back of her head that required several stitches. Still, she insisted that she was perfectly safe to live alone and had no intention of moving or allowing anyone to move in with her. And although the family worried about her, they acknowledged that her independence was important and so tried to respect her wishes, checking on her daily and doing what they could to support her solitary living situation.

One day, Gail, her daughter, received a call from a neighbor. Mrs. Isaacson had apparently fallen in the back yard and lain on the wet grass in the rain for several hours before she was discovered. She was hospitalized for hypothermia and dehydration but was expected to recover, albeit weaker than before. During the

T. A. Harvath, M. Fedyk, *What If Maslow Was Wrong?*,
https://doi.org/10.1007/978-3-032-14249-8_2

hospitalization, her children decided that this was the last straw and that their mother was no longer safe to live alone. They half joked about the newspaper running a story of how a "crazy cat lady" was found dead in her yard and that the family would be vilified for doing nothing to help her. Reluctantly, they arranged for her to be transferred to an assisted living facility that specialized in memory care when she was discharged from the hospital.

When she realized she was in "an old folks' home," Mrs. Isaacson was livid and determined to find a way out. She was agitated and combative and, initially, refused to cooperate with any of the care the staff tried to provide. After about a week, she calmed down and no longer fought with the staff, though she continued to beg to be taken home whenever the family visited. She also figured out that if you knew the code you could leave the locked facility. Try as she might, she was not able to escape, but it didn't stop her from trying!

One day, Gail received a call from the facility informing her that another resident had come into Mrs. Isaacson's room and the two had an altercation. The other resident hit Mrs. Isaacson over the head with his cane, resulting in a visible contusion and a small laceration over her left eye. Despite unanimous, vehement family objections and written advance directives that indicated no invasive interventions were to be implemented, the ALF insisted on sending Mrs. Isaacson to the emergency department of the local hospital for a CT scan of her head. The family argued that it didn't matter what was found; she was not a candidate for surgical intervention. Still, the administrator insisted it "was for her own safety."

Predictably, Mrs. Isaacson refused to cooperate with the CT scan and started to demand that she be sent home instead of being returned to the ALF. After several hours of coaxing and gentle persuasion, Mrs. Isaacson was returned to the ALF, having refused all medical intervention in the emergency department. She suffered no discernable long-term ill effects from the fall and quickly returned to her usual daily routine of standing near the exit, hoping to follow someone out.

Several weeks later, Gail got another call from the ALF administrator informing her that Mrs. Isaacson had been involved in yet another altercation with a resident who entered her room uninvited. This time, a staff member witnessed the other resident shove her to the floor resulting in a fracture to her right hip. Again, she was transported to the emergency department; this time, she was admitted because return to the memory care unit was not an option.

Not surprisingly, this hospitalization was the beginning of a downward spiral for Mrs. Isaacson. It started with pneumonia that was likely related to immobility and then progressed to "failure to thrive." Two weeks after her fracture, Mrs. Isaacson was admitted to a nursing home for hospice care. She died 3 weeks later. At her funeral, her family could not help but wonder whether they had made the right decision in removing her from her home. While they had rightly been concerned about her safety, they were dismayed to admit that the congregate care environment had not been able to provide her with the safeguards they were seeking.

2.2 Chapter Outline

Mrs. Isaacson's situation illustrates many of the challenges that can arise when family and healthcare professionals intervene to "protect" the older adult with dementia. While these efforts often reflect the best of intentions, undesirable consequences are all too common. In examining the tension between concerns for the safety of individuals with dementia and respect for their expressed preferences or autonomy, it is important to recognize that the word "safety" has a variety of meanings. This chapter explores some of the different meanings of the word "safety," with a particular focus one how these meanings intersect with concerns about the quality of life for older adults. Unfortunately, none of the most common ways of defining safety in healthcare are useful for figuring out how to protect someone's safety unless you also ask, "Ok, what kind of system are we thinking about here?" The reason is that, as Maslow points out, there is no such thing as safety in complete isolation from society (Maslow 1943). Maslow stressed: "It is too often not realized that culture itself is an adaptive tool, one of whose main functions is to make the physiological emergencies come less and less often" (Maslow 1943, page 377).

We build many different systems for living in our social world—our churches, our schools, our houses, and our hospitals. One of the functions of these systems is to keep us safe. To understand what safety means in Mrs. Isaacson's case, we must compare the two "safety-generating social systems" that are at the heart of her case, her home filled with stray cats, and the ALF where she spent the last months of her life. Perhaps surprisingly, if we compare these two systems to nuclear reactors and air travel, we will get to several important insights about what safety means for patients like Mrs. Isaacson.

2.3 Safety as Error Reduction

Probably the most common concept of safety currently in use in nursing and medicine is a concept that is usually expressed with the phrase "patient safety." This in turn is often linked to efforts to actively reduce clinical errors. In the landmark publication, *To Err Is Human* (Institute of Medicine (US) Committee on Quality of Health Care in America 2000), it was noted that up to 98,000 deaths each year in the United States could be attributed to preventable medical errors. The cost of those errors, both in terms of human lives and in real dollars, provided incentive to focus much needed attention on the reduction of medical errors. Since the publication of *To Err Is Human*, massive efforts at local, state, and national levels have been directed toward preventing or eliminating medical errors that contribute to poor outcomes for patients who are recipients of healthcare in this country. What all these efforts have in common is that they try to implement standardized systems within hospitals, clinics, memory care facilities, and so on. Teams and departments within each system are charged with tracking those systems so that the points at which failures of safety emerge can be monitored.

An unintended consequence of this evolution in how healthcare-related safety-generated social spaces are configured has been the growing perception among patients, families, and lay audiences that all medical errors can and should be prevented—we just need to invest more time and energy into engineering clinical spaces and training the staff so that there are checks and processes in place that will be effective in preventing all but the most extreme risks. In fact, there is an (unspoken) assumption in healthcare education programs that it is not only desirable but possible to create error-free healthcare.

But this is an impossible goal, as we will explain in more details below. For now, here is a simple example that helps warm you up to our deeper point. When Terri was working as a clinical nurse specialist in a veterans' nursing home, the management of the nursing home implemented a barcode medication administration system. They quickly learned that the nursing staff administered over 10,000 doses of medications each month. Now, think about doing something very simple like writing out your full name or filling a glass of water. Could you do either of these things without ever, due to boredom or fatigue, getting a letter wrong or spilling a drop of water? It really is not possible to do something 10,000 times in a row without making a mistake. Even the most automated and expensive of industrial processes do not aspire to error-free systems. The famous "six-sigma" process for quality control tries to reduce error to just 3.4 per million operations, and it applies only to fully automated, almost entirely human-free manufacturing systems.

The point is that safety as error reduction does not mean safety as complete error elimination; and safety as error reduction requires investing a lot of time and energy making the environment as visible and standardized as possible.

2.4 Safety as Liability Reduction

Sometimes, we use the term "safety" when what we mean is liability reduction: a clinic is safe only when it will be extremely hard for its patients to successfully sue either the providers who work at the clinic or the management of the clinic for things that can happen at the clinic. When we are using this concept, we talk about "protecting" patients when in fact what we mean is protecting institutions or providers from lawsuits.

A number of studies have demonstrated that some of the best safeguards against malpractice litigation include developing positive relationships with the patient and family and engaging in open and honest communication (Wojcieszak et al. 2007; Stelfox et al. 2005). But these practices don't actually protect patients and don't necessarily result in fewer errors. Instead of apologies, what often happens is that a system responds by asserting that the care involved adhered to the "standard of care" that is delivered to every patient. In other words, the facility in charge of treating the patient treated the patient "as they would treat any other patient with the same medical needs and problems." This standard makes it very hard to include in the care plans for patients any of the patient's distinctive wishes or goals whenever these wishes or goals come into conflict with what is perceived to be the course of action which keeps liability risk as low as possible. While standards of care are important to ensure that clinicians are adhering to trusted and evidence-based practices, good clinical care also mandates that care be individualized to patients, given their circumstances and expressed preferences.

In the situation with Mrs. Isaacson, the ALF administrator insisted that she be sent to the emergency department (ED) when another resident struck her in the head with his cane "for her own safety." It is not clear how this intervention was supposed to enhance Mrs. Isaacson's safety: she had already been hit on her head! But the decision makes sense if "safety" means to reduce the risk of liability to the ALF. Getting hit on her head was out of the ALF's control, but sending Mrs. Isaacson to the ED was not, and doing the latter is exactly what a prudent clinical administrator would decide for almost any "typical patient." Perhaps the administrator was concerned that Mrs. Isaacson had sustained a serious head injury or was at risk for a subdural hematoma. At 101 years of age with progressive dementia, however, the risks involved in any surgical intervention were likely greater than any discernable benefit. Indeed, her daughter pleaded with the administrator that he not transport her mother to the ED, arguing that it would be too traumatic for her confused and frail mother and would not change the course of her care in any measurable way. In addition, it is important to note that Mrs. Isaacson had signed advanced directives on file that indicated that she was to have no resuscitative or invasive interventions but was to be "kept comfortable." Mrs. Isaacson was not just the "typical patient." She had expressed preferences that were ignored, presumably to protect the ALF, not Mrs. Isaacson!

Often, administrators and clinicians in healthcare settings will cite a policy as the reason for a given action, as if the policy was an inviolable law that was immutable. Healthcare policies are important tools designed by humans to try to ensure that evidence-based procedures and practices are clearly delineated so clinicians can provide care that adheres to the prevailing standard of care. And they can provide important protection from liability for a healthcare facility. However, policies, just like standards of care, cannot cover every individual patient situation and rely on each administrator's and each clinician's judgment when implemented. And policies, just like standards of care, can and should change over time to reflect our growing knowledge. Ironically, to argue that the ALF facility's policy is sufficient rationale to require Mrs. Isaacson to be transported to the ED given her other circumstances could actually increase the facility's liability by failing to implement person-centered care.

2.5 Safety as Taking Away the Freedom to Make Choices

Another meaning for "safety" that you will frequently find in healthcare settings turns the concept into an ethical rule that can be used to stop a person from making choices for themselves if that person's care team disagrees with those choices. For example, there were vending machines in one of the nursing homes where Terri worked. Some of the staff argued that nursing home residents should not be allowed to eat from the vending machines because the food choices are contraindicated for residents with diabetes or heart conditions. And, certainly, triple bypass patients probably don't need the fat, cholesterol, and calories that potato chips and cookies provide. However, Terri suspected that the nursing home staff didn't need the fat, cholesterol, and calories that potato chips and cookies provide either.

Of course, many people eat food that is bad for their health. However, as adults, we are allowed to make choices for ourselves, even if they are bad choices in terms of individual health—as long as they don't cause harm to others. In a free society, we are allowed to use whatever rules or standards we want to make our choices. We can carefully weigh the risks and benefits of a course of action. Or we can act only to satisfy our most immediate desires. Most of us fall somewhere in the middle: we may put a lot of thought into the most consequential of actions, like what kind of insurance provider to choose or what kind of truck to buy, but there is probably no one alive who has walked by a vending machine filled with salty and sweet snacks and has not at least been tempted! Either way, we are not required to provide reasons for all our choices. We recognize and accept that in pursuing our individual desires we sometimes take on risks or satisfy desires to enhance quality of life.

But sometimes when someone becomes old, frail, and demented, their caregivers start to make these kinds of decisions for them. The nurses, doctors, and family members who care for an older individual may start to consider increasingly restrictive sets of constraints—Should we take away the car keys? Should we do all the grocery shopping and menu planning? Should we move her into a memory-care facility?—that gradually put more weight on risk and harm reduction than prioritizing quality of life. Pushed to an extreme, caregivers may find themselves taking away all a person's choice because they are perceived as unsafe.

Mrs. Isaacson had lived in a marginally clean house for most of her adult life. She began taking in stray animals long before she developed dementia. And while her children frowned on this behavior for years, they would not have dreamed of interfering or forcefully removing the cats while their mother was still cognitively intact. Caring for the cats reflected a very deep choice about how Mrs. Isaacson wanted to live her life. As her dementia progressed, however, Mrs. Isaacson's children developed a stronger sense of responsibility: they wanted to "protect" their mother from the situation she had created as an adult with full decisional capacity (and perhaps they wanted to protect themselves from the judgment that might befall them if "the newspapers get ahold of this!"). We can convince ourselves that we have the right to prescribe the limits of another's freedom of choice if we do so under the banner of "promoting patient safety." A question to ask is "Does the change in Mrs. Isaacson's cognitive status give us the right to nullify decisions she made when she had capacity?"

2.6 Safety as Physical Harm Reduction

Finally, we sometimes use the term "safety" when we are, in fact, concerned about protecting patients from real or potential dangers. We think that this is the most useful concept of safety to use when thinking about how to care for older patients. But as with all the other concepts, some nuance is required when using.

The first nuance to understand is that this concept of safety is measurable because it is ultimately about whether certain actions or choices produce the intended effects, for example, while many clinicians believe that physical restrains can protect patients from harm, there is a tremendous amount of evidence that physical restraints sometimes cause more injuries than they prevent (see, for example, Cleary and Prescott 2015; Abraham et al. 2020).

But because this concept of safety is tied (pun intended) to the causal effect, it is tied to the environment—the "safety-generating social systems"—that we referred to above. Mrs. Isaacson's family had her transferred to an assisted living facility because they recognized she was no longer safe to live at home alone. They did this assuming the ALF would provide a measure of safety not possible in her home. But as we have already sadly observed, this was a false assumption: the injuries she sustained while living at the ALF ultimately lead to her death. This left the family wondering whether she might not have been better off staying in her own home, despite the risks. Indeed, from the perspective that safety means the ability to shield of a person from harmful causes and effects, it is not clear that the ALF was safer than Mrs. Isaacson's home. It has the appearance of safety, however, because some of the risks to Mrs. Isaacson's safety within the ALF were less salient to Mrs. Isaacson's family. They had no knowledge about how interactions between Mrs. Isaacson and other residents at the facility would go!

In nursing home settings, we have seen a proliferation of tab and wander alarm usage (Kiely et al. 2000; Aud 2004; Ali and Li 2016). We implement these "safeguards" to protect unrestrained patients from falling or from wandering into unsafe spaces. But despite the rapid advance in these technologies, residents in nursing home still are routinely injured from falls. The monitoring systems, though, give us the illusion of safety: just like we observed with the concept of safety as clinician error reduction, these technologies make the safety-generating social spaces that older adults live in more visible to staff and administrators. Because of this, clinicians can comfort themselves by thinking that at least they are doing *something* to try to prevent injuries. Family caregivers may join the clinicians in thinking this way and sometimes insist that restraints or alarms be used. But as a causal matter, a wander or tab alarm cannot prevent someone from falling. It just makes it easier for staff to know when a patient or resident has fallen and potentially injured themselves. But it does have real effects on the patient's quality of life. No one likes being monitored or observed by passive surveillance technology.

The cold, hard reality is that, at 101 years of age, Mrs. Isaacson had limited time left to live. Eventually, she was going to die. No one could say with 100% certainty that it would have been better for her to be at home than in the ALF. Had she stayed in her home she likely would have had greater quality of life than was provided to her in the ALF, but she also would have been exposed to an increasing number of rather obvious dangers.

What is clear, however, is that the ALF was not itself a perfectly safe environment. It tried to achieve safety through the four concepts of safety that we have listed. Staff were trained to minimize their errors, and the facility was clearly managed with an eye to reducing the threat of lawsuit; decisions were made that slowly stripped Mrs. Isaacson of her freedom of choice to prevent her from putting herself in harm's way, and many of these decisions were motivated by the belief that, by living in the ALF, Mrs. Isaacson would be safer because she would no longer be exposed to the risks of living at her home with stray cats and steps and doors to the outside that she could use at will. The decision to place Mrs. Isaacson in an ALF reflected her family's sincere belief it was in her best interest because it was the safest. The gift of hindsight helps us see that it was a decision that, like all too many of these kinds of decisions, was made without a thorough consideration of the risks that *each* option entailed and the impact of each decision on Mrs. Isaacson's quality of life.

2.7 Safety and Systems

Both the ALF and Mrs. Isaacson's house are safety-generating social systems. What this means is that each is "system" is configured to create a balance of the different kinds of safety we just reviewed or, since it is easier to think about, a different balance of the risks for each option. If we pretend that the appraisal of risks Mrs. Issacson was facing when her family was deciding where she would live can be measured on a scale running from 1 to 10, with 10 representing the highest risk, here is how these the appraisal of risks of the two living arrangements can be compared (see Table 2.1).

In contrast, if we examine the family's appraisal of risks of each choice after her death, a different picture emerges (see Table 2.2).

While these numbers are arbitrarily chosen, they do reflect the relative risks in Mrs. Isaacson's situation. Note that, in retrospect, the total risk of the ALF (21) is much higher than the total risk of her house (10). This means that while avoiding physical harms was the concept of safety that was most influential in decisions about her care, it was not appreciably different in the different settings. Because of this, we want to focus a bit of attention on how this concept of safety works, and this is where nuclear reactors and air travel come into the discussion.

2.8 Physical Harms and "Safety-Generating Social Systems"

The field of accident research was launched in the early 1980s, and some of its earliest work was inspired by the research of the sociologist Charles Perrow. He was interested in how societies adapted to incredibly complex technologies that can create catastrophic risks. He was one of the first scientists to analyze the partial meltdown of the nuclear reactor at Three Mile Island in 1979, and he also wrote about the risks of catastrophic physical harm inherent in air travel, genetic engineering, advanced weapons systems, and space missions (Perrow 1999). Perrow argued that there is no way of building a system of air travel (or any of the other systems he examined) capable of transporting millions of people without eventually experiencing what he called "normal accidents."

A normal accident is a by-product of the system itself. The accident is also predictable, that is to say, the specific, detailed way that the system fails itself won't be predictable, but the fact that the system will fail and cause some great physical harm *is* predictable. Perrow argues that these systems will fail because they are built with complex interactions that can cause unpredictable actions and because these interactions are built with tightly coupled interactions that can cause unintended chain reactions if one or more things go wrong. He called this property of the system its *interactive complexity*. If Perrow is right, it is almost impossible to build safety-generating social systems, including Mrs. Issacson's ALF, that won't eventually fail in some significant way because of interactive complexity.

Perrow notes that the nuclear reactors at Three Miles Island were built with a complex system of valves and sensors for moving both radioactive and nonradioactive water around the reactor cores. Because the two kinds of water were drawn from the same (nonradioactive) source and because water can flow backward through any pipe if a valve breaks, it was possible for the flow of water through the whole reactor system to follow patterns that had never been predicted or anticipated by the engineers who designed the reactor. Simplifying tremendously, it was the failure of a single sensor and a single valve that caused the water in the no. 2 reactor at Three Mile Island to flow through the cooling system in a way that the reactor operators could neither observe nor understand, preventing them from making informed operational decisions that would ensure the reactor could not meltdown. Perrow argues that, through luck, a complete meltdown was avoided (some operators made good guesses about the movement and temperature of the water once they realized something was wrong); if they had made different guesses, then the accident would have been much, much more costly and harmful.

But interactive complexity alone isn't the cause of normal accidents. *Tight coupling* is the other concept that we need to understand. If you have ever visited the DMV or just about any modern hospital, you have already experienced a tightly coupled social system. In a tightly coupled social system, there are chains of cause and effect that are rigidly sequenced with very little opportunity for intervention in the case of failure. At the DMV, there is only one process for getting your license, and it involves filling out this form, then this form, and then this form and then taking this test; and if any step isn't completed the right way, then you must start over. Air travel is another example of a tightly coupled system: if you don't make the gate on time, the plane will leave without you; there are so many parts to the system that have to move in harmony with one another that even the smallest deviation—a plane waiting an extra 10 min for a family that cannot get across the airport in time to make their connection—could cause the whole system to break down.

When a system with interactive complexity and tight coupling causes harm, it is often because of its ability to generate nonlinear effects. What that means is that something very small—the failure of a single sensor—can generate a cascading sequence of cause and effects that eventually leads to catastrophe.

In the air travel example, we can often wonder why a plane won't wait for a family with small children to run across an airport to catch their connecting flight. When, however, we understand that planes are given tight windows to keep their place in the queues for takeoffs and landings and if they miss that place in the queue and their landing is delayed, that means that passengers on that plane will miss their tight connections and so on; we can begin to understand how that brief wait can cause a chain reaction of delays that magnify the outcomes for many more passengers than just that one family. When we add weather delays, unexpected mechanical problems, or delays of incoming flight crews, perhaps we can appreciate that a system that is so complex and tightly coupled can't always be responsive to the needs of a small number of passengers. Social systems with high levels of interactive complexity and tight coupling often cannot be highly responsive to the needs or values of the individuals who have to interact with the system.

2.9 Mrs. Issacson's ALF

As we've seen, Mrs. Isaacson's family was probably most concerned with her physical safety, especially as her cognitive status and decisional capacity began to deteriorate. This makes sense, anyway, of their choice to move her into the ALF. But as the two accidents that Mrs. Isaacson suffered while she was in the ALF show, the ALF has the characteristics of a tightly coupled system with high levels of interactive complexity. Interactions between residents are inevitable; this is interactive complexity. And the staff and management's concerns about legal liability force them to respond to adverse interactions between residents in a way that tightly couples their reactions to the adverse interactions. In short, we have a system in which "normal accidents" are inevitable: catastrophic harms will occur simply as a matter of time.

This is not to argue that Mrs. Isaacson would have been safer if she had remained in her home, living with her cats. Rather, the point is that, had an accident occurred, it would have been a different kind of accident: it seems like very few things in Mrs. Isaacson's home were tightly coupled. After all, when she fell in her backyard, she had sadly remained there for several hours. This would not be possible in the ALF.

The conclusion we want to leave you with, then, is that even when we go out of our way to design nursing homes or hospitals to be as safe as possible—even when we invest years of research and training—we may end up building a unique kind of risk. Because ALFs usually have the characteristics of interactive complexity and tightly coupled processes, "normal accidents" at ALFs are predictable. This is not to say that the ALF staff could have predicted that Mrs. Isaacson was going to be struck or shoved. Rather, it is important to understand that ALFs (and all complex systems) carry risks. They should not be seen as a risk-free alternative to

Table 2.1 Family appraisal of potential risks for Mrs. Isaacson prior to placement

	ALF	Mrs. Isaacson's house
Risk of medical error	5	2
Risk of lawsuit for Mrs. Isaacson	0	1
Risk of loss of choice	8	0
Risk of physical harm	1	9

Table 2.2 Family appraisal of potential risks for Mrs. Isaacson after her death

	ALF	Mrs. Isaacson's house
Risk of medical error	5	2
Risk of lawsuit for Mrs. Isaacson	0	1
Risk of loss of choice	8	0
Risk of physical harm	8	7

home-based living situations. At best, they offer a different balance of risks than in the home. When families are deciding whether to place an older family member in a congregate care environment, they should be apprised of the risks for *each* option, at least to the best of our knowledge. That broadens the decision-making to include the other kinds of risks to safety. In Tables 2.1 and 2.2, it is important to note that while the appraisal of risk to physical safety was not substantially different in home versus ALF, the risk to choice was substantial. Had Mrs. Isaacson's family been privy to a more nuanced understanding of the risks to safety and the trade-offs, they may still have chosen ALF placement. If, however, they had understood that the ALF carried its own risks for their mother's physical safety, they might not have second-guessed their decision.

Discussion and Reflection Questions

1. Imagine a time in the distant future when you might have some significant health issues. If your primary care provider told you that you were no longer safe to drive, how would you respond? If your family suggested that you were no longer safe to live in your own home, what would your reaction be? What if their assessment of your abilities was much lower than your own? How would you feel being told you must now accept help?
2. This chapter introduces some of the meanings of "safety" as the concept is used in healthcare, including error reduction, liability reduction, taking away choice, and physical harm reduction. How do these different interpretations of safety conflict or align in real-world geriatric care scenarios? How might understanding these distinctions impact your approach to patient care in the future?
3. The case of Mrs. Isaacson highlights the tension between ensuring an older adult's safety and respecting their autonomy and quality of life. In your future

practice, how will you navigate situations where a patient's choices might introduce risks, and what strategies can you employ to balance their independence with concerns for their well-being?

4. The chapter introduces the idea that different environments (like a home vs. an ALF) are "safety-generating social systems" with inherent risks that can be traced back to how these "systems" are engineered. How does understanding the concepts of interactive complexity and tight coupling influence your perception of safety in various care settings for older adults? What do these concepts imply about the ability of the ALF to be responsive to the individual values of patient like Mrs. Isaacson?
5. The concept of "normal accidents" suggests that failures are predictable in complex, tightly coupled systems. How does this idea challenge the notion that all risks can be eliminated in geriatric care? What are the ethical implications of accepting that some accidents may be "normal" in certain care systems, and how should this influence decision-making for patients and their families?

References

Abraham J, Hirt J, Kamm F, Möhler R (2020) Interventions to reduce physical restraints in general hospital settings: a scoping review of components and characteristics. J Clin Nurs 29(17–18):3183–3200

Ali H, Li H (2016) Designing a smart watch interface for a notification and communication system for nursing homes. In: Human aspects of IT for the aged population. Design for aging, Lecture notes in computer science. Springer International Publishing, Cham, pp 401–411

Aud MA (2004) Dangerous wandering: elopements of older adults with dementia from long-term care facilities. Am J Alzheimers Dis Other Dement 19(6):361–368

Cleary K, Prescott K (2015) The use of physical restraints in acute and long-term care: an updated review of the evidence, regulations, ethics, and legality. J Acute Care Phys Ther 6(April):8–15

Institute of Medicine (US) Committee on Quality of Health Care in America (2000) To err is human: building a safer health system. National Academies Press (US), Washington

Kiely DK, Morris JN, Algase DL (2000) Resident characteristics associated with wandering in nursing homes. Int J Geriatr Psychiatry 15(11):1013–1020

Maslow AH (1943) A theory of human motivation. Psychol Rev 50(4):370–396

Perrow C (1999) Normal accidents: living with high risk technologies - updated edition. Princeton University Press, Princeton

Stelfox HT, Gandhi TK, Orav EJ, Gustafson ML (2005) The relation of patient satisfaction with complaints against physicians and malpractice lawsuits. Am J Med 118(10):1126–1133

Wojcieszak D, Saxton JW, Finkelstein MM (2007) Sorry works!: disclosure, apology, and relationships prevent medical malpractice claims. AuthorHouse

Impossible Choices and Cost-Benefit Analysis

3

3.1 Case Illustration

Victoria Callahan was an 83-year-old woman who was terminally ill following a 6-year battle with cancer of the jaw. Prior to her cancer diagnosis, Dr. Callahan, a doctorally prepared nurse, was very active and engaged in her community and in professional organizations. Friends and colleagues often sought her advice on complex matters on a wide range of topics, and she served on numerous boards and committees.

When she was first diagnosed with cancer, she underwent major surgery and radiation treatments. Unfortunately, she experienced multiple, serious complications over the course of her illness journey (e.g., *infections, osteomyelitis,* etc.*) requiring frequent hospitalizations, repeated hyperbaric oxygen treatments, and multiple surgeries. Throughout all these challenges, Dr. Callahan maintained a clear understanding of her prognosis and openly discussed her preferences for end-of-life care. She had advanced directives indicating she did not want resuscitation or ventilation if her heart stopped or she stopped breathing. She also had additional written instructions that clearly stated that she did not want to be kept alive if her health condition prevented her from engaging in a meaningful life. She defined "meaningful life" as being able to engage in in-depth conversations with others and remain active in her community.*

Approximately 5 months prior to her death, Dr. Callahan was facing a challenging healthcare decision. She had a bone fragment poking through her cheek into her mouth that caused sharp pain every time she spoke. Her surgeon was advocating for an invasive surgery to rebuild her jaw, believing he could restore her oral function while providing a better cosmetic look to her face. She was reluctant to undergo this surgery because the years of cancer, its treatments, and complications had left her quite frail. She sought the counsel of close friends and family to help her with the decision. She asked them to get a white board so that she could see each option and the pros/cons of those options and the likelihood the option would restore/maintain her quality of life (*see* Table 3.1).

T. A. Harvath, M. Fedyk, *What If Maslow Was Wrong?*,
https://doi.org/10.1007/978-3-032-14249-8_3

Table 3.1 Dr. Callahan's cost-benefit analysis

Option	Pros	Cons	Quality of life
No surgery, comfort measures only	Given her frailty, this would not put her at risk for further complications	She could not speak comfortably. Was "comfort" possible?	Not being able to speak was frustrating. Speaking was painful. She was unable to write quickly enough to communicate as she wanted with others
Aid in dying (she lived in a place where this was legal)	This would allow her a measure of control	She didn't feel she was "done" with her work with others and in her community	This would allow her to escape the constant pain she was experiencing and avoid a dying process where she might lose control
Minimally invasive surgery to clip the bone	This might ease the pain and allow her to continue with some of her activities	Because of all the radiation and her frailty, she was not a good surgical candidate. It was not clear that her wounds would heal from even minor surgery	This option offered her some hope that her quality of life might be restored to a level that was satisfactory for her
More invasive surgery to repair the jaw, using a flap from her deltoid to heal the tissue	This might provide even greater pain relief that would allow her to eat and speak with ease	A more invasive surgery carried more risks of complications and a recovery course that would likely be arduous	While this option offered her hope for a quality of life she valued, the cosmetic improvements were not important to her, and her history of postsurgical complications made this option less desirable

After careful consideration of these options, she decided to try the minimally invasive surgery. She believed that the potential for better quality of life with less pain was worth the risk. She understood that although she would have a tracheostomy following surgery because of the swelling, she was clear that she did not want long-term ventilation if there were complications.

3.2 Surrogate Decision-Making and the Wisdom of Dr. Callahan

Most persons are not like Dr. Callahan. They do not write out the cost and benefits of each course of treatment and then analyze the different choices using constraints that are derived from their values. Instead, many persons—or the family members of persons—use a single, and usually very simple, rule to make end-of-life decisions. One of the most popular single rules that clinicians hear from family members is "Do everything!". Another very popular single rule is "We don't want her to feel any pain" or the close variation "We just want him to be comfortable." Another very popular single rule is "We just want our mother to be safe!". Using a single rule makes a certain amount of sense. It cuts down on both the initial amount of uncertainty and—important when someone is facing a stressful, complicated choice—mental effort required to figure out what to do. These are important benefits when facing an impossible choice.

While these are helpful rules, end-of-life decision-making is extremely complex, and there is a lot of uncertainty inherent to the process. Our goal in this chapter is to try to show you the wisdom of thinking like Dr. Callahan. When facing an impossible choice, it can be helpful to write out a table that describes the risks and benefits of different courses of action. This is helpful not only because it provides persons and their family members with an opportunity to reflect on their values in some detail. The table itself can be a helpful source of information for clinicians and family members to make decisions from in case it is no longer possible to communicate with the person. Some of you may be thinking that this cost-benefit analysis is already built into the process for obtaining consent for surgery or other interventions that involve some measure of risk. It is important to remember, however, that the potential risks and benefits spelled out in a consent form are generalized for the intervention, not for the individual person. The type of cost-benefit analysis we are referring to is individualized to the older adult, taking account their preferences, their ideas about what constitutes quality of life, and the potential risks that are particularly salient to their situation.

Again, our aim is to gently suggest that, even though it is messier than following a single rule like "Just keep Mum safe!", working with the key concepts for this chapter and building a cost-benefit table just like Dr. Callahan can be a more practical way of helping to make things just a little better when caring for someone at the end of their life.

3.3 Substituted Judgment

Situations involving substituted judgment arise whenever a person lacks the capacity (either temporarily or permanently) to make decisions on their own behalf. A father of an adult child might have to make medical decisions for his son if his son has been in a car accident that left him unconscious or if an adult daughter needs to make decisions on behalf of her mother who is experiencing an episode of delirium that is impairing her mother's decisional capacity. In these situations, one person is making decisions *for* another person, and these decisions count as *substituted judgments* when the person making the decisions on behalf of a person makes the decision that the *person him or herself would make*. From an ethical standpoint, it is important for the person making substituted judgments not to make decisions about what is best for *them* or what *they* want for their son or their mother or their cousin or their wife but, instead, to make the decision their son, mother, cousin, or wife would make for themselves were they capable of making decisions on their own. In order to make that decision, the person providing the substituted judgment needs to have a reasonable understanding of what the person with diminished decisional capacity would want—but often, they don't.

That is an important point. We have both seen families trapped in making decisions about end-of-life care where the family oscillates between making decisions that are based in avoiding fights among family members on the one hand and making decisions that reflect what their family member would want on the other hand. It is quite difficult to make substituted judgments on behalf of another person[1] when there are pressures to make decisions designed to satisfy the needs of family members, especially when it is impossible for anyone to know whether the decision that you make really is a bona fide substituted judgment or just a lucky coincidence between what the person would want and what the family members want.

When clinicians think about situations where an older adult's family member must make a substituted judgment on behalf of the older adult and this family member also faces pressures from their own desires or the emotions of other family members to make any number of different decisions, it is important to consider a principle that is foundational to the ethical training that all clinicians receive. The principle is called the *principle of autonomy*, and it means no decision about a person's care is ethically justified unless it can be tied directly to knowledge of what a person wants or values *for themselves*. In the context of care for older adults, this principle is often referred to as *person-centered care*. It means making sure that all clinical activities and operations are organized so that they do not prevent a person from expressing "what they want for themselves" and so that a person can not only consent but also, ideally, help shape or direct any significant medical or clinical intervention. (We'll return to these principles again in much greater detail in later chapters).

From the clinician's perspective, cases involving substituted judgment can seem risky. It is hard for clinicians to ensure that they are living up to the duty of providing person-centered care if the family member making decisions on behalf of a person is really making decisions that are designed to appease family members who are stressed out or afraid about what is going to happen to the older adult. At the same time, it is hard for a family member who is making substituted decisions on behalf of a person to *prove* that they really are making decisions, as best they can, in a way that reflects what the older adult herself would have wanted. We have both seen many cases in which communication breaks down between a family and a care team because neither side has enough trust that each is making decisions "the right way." The care team may doubt that the family is making decisions that are consistent with the duties of person-centered care; conversely, the family may believe that the care team is treating the older adult just like any other older adult, not taking into consideration the older adult's values or preferences. And sometimes the family dynamics are just messy, for example, Terri worked with a family of an older man

[1] It is worth noting that we avoid using the phrase "loved one" when referring to family members or friends in these situations. This is based on a recognition that not all families share love, even if they are involved in caregiving. We believe it is important to understand that surrogate decision-makers don't necessarily make substituted judgments from a place of love.

who had clear advance directives. His choice was to be allowed to die in comfort if his heart or lungs stopped. He designated his daughter as his surrogate decision-maker because he knew it would be hard for his wife to make the decision to withhold life-sustaining treatments. When his health deteriorated, his daughter struggled to make the decisions she knew her father wanted because she could see the impact they would have on her mother.

It is in situations like this that the table that Dr. Callahan made can be quite helpful. Of course, Dr. Callahan was able to fill the table on her own. But what we are suggesting is that, in cases where a need for substituted judgment arises, the family and the care team can sit down together and fill out the table of risks and benefits together. This gives the family the time and the means to weave the values and preferences of the older adult into the logical structure of the clinical decisions that the older adult is facing. And it can reassure the clinicians that the family members are really expressing substituted judgments on behalf of the persons. Working on the table together can prevent breakdowns in trust and communication.

We think this is an important practical benefit. It means that both family members and providers might need to set aside more time to analyze the costs, benefits, and impacts on quality of life of a decision. But it also ensures that persons, families, and providers are making decisions together.

3.4 The Best-Interest Standard

At this point, the following question has probably occurred to you, "OK—I see the value of filling in a table like Dr. Callahan. That is a good idea—but what should I do if I just don't know what the older person wants or values? How am I supposed to make that decision if I am not allowed to just substitute what *I* want or what another family member *wants*?" It is at this point that we can introduce another decision-making aid, the best-interest standard.

The best-interest standard is one of the oldest ideas in medical decision-making, and it can sometimes be difficult to apply (Baumrucker et al. 2008; Diekema 2011; Kopelman 1997). But its core intuition is straightforward even if a bit wordy: when you don't know what a specific person's wishes, values, or preferences are about a specific medical treatment, intervention, or clinical decision, then, rather than trying to guess at what *they* would want, try to evaluate the treatment, intervention, or decision by determining what outcomes the choice can impact, where these outcomes are outcomes that almost anyone would value. Put more simply, if you do not and cannot know a person's values, it is OK to assume that they care about minimizing pain (because most people care about minimizing pain), that they care about preserving their dignity (because most people care about preserving dignity), or that they care about being cared for and avoiding a situation in which some of their needs are neglected (because most people care about being cared for and not having their needs neglected) or anything else. The best-interest standard allows us to fill in gaps in our knowledge of a person's values with commonly held values.

What this means is that the best-interest standard can be used to fill in a decision-making table like Dr. Callahan's. In fact, some of Dr. Callahan's preferences and values align with the values that can be used when making decisions according to the best-interest standard, values like being able to communicate and having her dignity preserved. You can imagine similar situations, then, where if Dr. Callahan had not been able to communicate her values and her caregivers did not know enough about Dr. Callahan's values to be able to express substituted judgment, reasoning from the best-interest standard would have generated similar information.

It can be tempting to assume that, in general, all humans share the *same* values: comfort, family, life, etc. That would be incorrect. We have likely all encountered individuals whose values are different from our own, for example, we have seen people with cancer who would rather endure some pain than experience the haze of narcotic pain medications. Or older adults who are frail and sick who, despite our inability to understand what quality of life they may have, still wish to be full codes and receive maximal efforts to remain alive. So, what should we do when a person has values that are not values that most people care about, at least not that specifically? Dr. Callahan placed value on the work that she was doing and cared that she be able to complete projects that were still ongoing. This may not be a value that is easy to generate using best-interest reasoning.

3.5 Advanced Directives

This challenge brings us to our next topic, the importance of advanced directives. In their simplest form, these can be tables like Dr. Callahan's that are prepared well in advance of any medical crisis. In fact, we both prepared our advanced directives when we were in our 40s and in good health. But they usually contain much more information that is useful to clinicians than Dr. Callahan's table, and because they are prepared in advanced, they can only make broad assumptions about what specific medical or clinical conditions a person could face.

The most common information in an advanced directive is an expression of preferences about what a person wants if they are unable to communicate their own wishes and either their heart or their breathing has stopped. The latter do not in fact mean that the person is beyond any medical intervention: chest compressions can restart a stopped heart, and a ventilator can be used to breath for a person if their lungs are unable to breath for them. But both interventions—and many like them, like the defibrillator, which uses electrical shocks to attempt to reset a stopped heart—are aggressive forms of treatment. Chest compressions can break ribs, and ventilators may require a patient to be sedated so they don't remove the breathing tube. But the most difficult aspect of these treatments is that, even if clinicians succeed in restarting a person's heart or restoring respiration, this usually does not mean that the person will soon get up out of bed and walk out of the hospital and return to the same level of function they had prior to the hospitalization. It is very common for persons who need these kinds of interventions to require ongoing, sometimes permanent, support. The data here is very complicated, but a recent

American Heart Association study found that roughly 25% of persons who required CPR while in the hospital survived and were able to leave the hospital (Sawyer et al. 2020).

So, the most common kind of information in an advanced directive is what is called "DNR/DNI" status, which stands for "do not resuscitate/do not intubate." Most states have prepared information packets about advanced directives that help people fill out the appropriate DNR/DNI preferences, and some states even pay for clinicians—usually nurses or social workers—to provide advice and consultation when filling out an advanced directive.

As we hope you can appreciate, advanced directives reduce some of the uncertainty that clinicians face when trying to provide person-centered care: a well-constructed advanced directive gives a clinical care team very specific guidance about how to treat a person in a way that protects the person's autonomy even if the person cannot speak and no family members are available to act as surrogate decision-makers.

But a typical advanced directive is often limited in its utility for situations like Dr. Callahan's. Dr. Callahan had to make some very specific decisions—impossible choices—about difficult courses of treatment. However, the total number of impossible choices was reduced because she also had an advanced directive that she had prepared years prior that elaborated on her values related to autonomy and quality of life. In practical terms, this meant that her risk-benefit table could be tailored to address those issues that were of particular importance to her, individually.

So, Dr. Callhan's table plus a well-designed advanced directive (see Appendix A for a copy of Terri's additional instructions to her advanced directives) would make substituted decision-making much easier and the need to rely on best-interest considerations much less likely. This is not the case, however, for a single-rule decision-making. A rule like "Just keep my mother comfortable!" does not tell clinicians what kind of surgical interventions are congruent with the person's values, and a rule like "Do everything!" does not consider the fact that all medical decisions involve mutually exclusive trade-offs. The point is that both rules breakdown and create even more decisional uncertainty than otherwise would be the case—leading to situations where substitute decision-making or best-interest reasoning must be relied upon.

But we also want to return to the big idea in this book: quality of life usually matters *more* than safety—especially if "safety" means "kept alive by any means necessary." We've explored several of the ways in which trying to prioritize safety can undermine quality of life, so we hope you will take that idea as established. Here, there is a more nuanced point. As a person nears the end of their life, there is less time and less energy available to make choices—to express one's agency—and so it is helpful to think of people as having a "savings account" of agency that they can spend a little from every day. Our suggestion here is to be aware of whether most of the spending from the agency savings account are spent on actions and choices meant to preserve safety—as opposed to actions that contribute to quality of life. In our clinical experience, we've both seen examples of the latter that range from delaying a treatment to attend a family wedding to sailing to England one last time. And in fact, in both cases, members of the care team opposed the person's decision on grounds of safety. In the first case, the palliative care team argued that delaying palliative radiation would reduce its effectiveness, and in the second case, being aboard a boat would make it too hard to get critical medical care if complications from a series of surgeries arose. In each case, the individual's expressed preferences were honored because they maintained decisional capacity.

3.6 Daily Decision-Making

We wanted to shift focus slightly here to share with you some thoughts about how to make decisions that are more routine, more day-to-day—like whether to have a bath or a shower—than high-stakes decisions, like whether to proceed with the surgery that Dr. Callahan was forced to consider, because ordinary life is filled with decisions and we don't want to suggest that it is possible or desirable to stop and construct a risk-benefit table like Dr. Callahan's every time a decision must be made. At the same time, toward the end of life, even the most mundane decisions can take on increased importance, for example, Dr. Callahan remained very particular about how her hair was combed, even as her capabilities diminished. These decisions, while day to day, do have increased meaning and moral significance.

The first observation we want to offer about these kinds of decisions is that we believe that quality of life never ceases to matter, no matter how serious the illness or how diminished someone's capacities become or how seemingly trivial the decision. Decision-making itself can be a way of recognizing—indeed, investing time and energy in—the activities and interpersonal engagements that provide life with its meaning and thus can be, for many people, one of the most important ways of protecting quality of life.

Another way of putting this point is that living never truly *ends*, even though life itself, for all of us, does eventually stop. There is no transition period where living is done, but someone is still alive and yet they are nevertheless unable to have their values or preferences realized or respected. Not even the more serious terminal diagnosis prevents someone from thinking like Dr. Callahan, about the ways in which life can still have meaning. Anyone who has tried to force an older adult with dementia to take a shower knows that even if we lack decisional capacity we are often able to communicate our preferences about how our daily life unfolds. Knowing that the end is near does not strip a person of their agency, and it does not require that they abandon all their personal values and beliefs, trading them in just for an overriding concern for safety.

3.7 Patterns of Life

Of course, you might want to object to our perspective on the importance of agency in the final years, months, weeks, days, or even hours of living. What if a person has suffered an injury—such as a stroke—that prevents them from having any conscious experience? And what should be done if that person also lacks a friend or family member who can act as their surrogate decision-maker? Yes, the care team can start making medical decisions on behalf of this person using the best-interest standard, but the logic of the best-interest decision-making only applies to serious medical questions. What about the rest of the decisions that must be made on behalf of such a person? How can we provide for such a person something that supports this person's agency regarding quality of life?

Here is an idea that we hope you might find helpful. Each of our lives contains any number of patterns and habits. Not all these patterns are healthy—for example, one of us enjoys cheesy popcorn way too much to keep a bag of it at home (well, actually, both of us enjoy cheesy popcorn!). But even these unhealthy habits reveal something important about a person's values: the patterns and habits in a person's life tend to *reflect* their values. A person who frequently goes on long hikes almost certainly values nature; a person who volunteers in a science museum almost certainly values teaching about biology and physics; a person who spends hours of the day talking to her daughters almost certainly values her family.

But an important thing about these patterns is that not only do they reveal a person's values—which of course they do!—but that they are almost always visible features of a person's life. It is relatively straightforward to find evidence from multiple different people about any of a person's most persistent patterns. With a little bit of detective work, it is possible to learn about the values of a person who is otherwise so ill that they cannot communicate or express their own wishes. Then, knowledge of these values can be a source of insight into how to ensure that there is still *quality* to a person's life despite the seriousness of their situation.

3.8 Durability of Preferences

There is one last idea we want to offer you before concluding this chapter. This is what is sometimes called the problem of the durability of preferences. It is an easy problem to grasp but can be quite gnarly in practice. In situations where older adults lack decisional capacity (e.g., in advanced dementia) and either do not have advanced directives or their advanced directives don't address the specific situation at hand, it may still be possible to discern what their preference might be. A growing body of research suggests that older adults with dementia may remain capable to participate in making some decisions related to their health and care. Some authors (Lahey and Elwyn 2020; Mellgard and Gligorov 2022) suggest that older adults with dementia be assessed not for decisional capacity per se but for their capacity to participate in specific decisions. This recognizes that decisions vary both in their complexity and in the severity of the consequences for different choices. Creating a "sliding scale" for individuals with dementia is a way to ensure their autonomy is maximized to the extent possible.

Research by Whitlatch and others (see, for example, Menne and Whitlatch 2007; Miller et al. 2016) have found that older adults with dementia are still able to communicate their likes and dislikes and that participation in decision-making adds to their quality of life. These expressions of preferences should not be discounted or dismissed simply because the person has dementia or lacks decisional capacity. Instead, they need to be part of the consideration given when decisions must be made. This is especially important for those everyday decisions such as the following: Do you want a shower or bath? Are you ready to get out of bed?

Does this mean that our choices and preferences, especially regarding advanced directives, are unchanging? No. We've already shared that both of your authors filled out their advanced directives in their 40s. Should a care team really feel that they are bounded by the specific DNR/DNI instructions written 40 years ago but never revisited if neither of us—thankfully!—are hospitalized with any serious conditions until we are in our late 80s? So, while patterns in a person life do reveal values and preferences, we should not also assume that preferences and values are so durable and static that they are unchanging. It is reasonable to ask whether four decades might be just too long of a time to be sure that a person's wishes for their care have not changed? Yes, which means that it is probably a good idea to refresh or revise your advanced directive every 5–10 years or when your life or your health or other conditions change.

But there is a more specific concern that we want to focus on: What happens when, in the context of dementia or delirium, the older adult's expression of preferences changes dramatically? This brings us back to Dr. Callahan.

3.9 Back to the Case

As her illness progressed, Dr. Callahan learned more about her specific situation and what the meaning of different risks to her would be. Both her advanced care planning and her ongoing care were, as clinicians would say, "person-centered." And until the very end, Dr. Callahan never lost her agency as her illness progressed. This allowed her, crucially, to change her mind—to express different values and preferences as the facts of her illness emerged and became known. Unfortunately, the surgery did not go as planned. Following surgery, she developed delirium and was confused and agitated at times. She resisted the daily care of her tracheostomy and slapped at the nurses who tried to do dressing changes on her surgical incision. After a few weeks, it was also clear that the effects of multiple courses of radiation therapy to her jaw meant that the skin flap failed and her surgical wound would likely never heal. Because Dr. Callahan now lacked decisional capacity, the care team, in conversation with Dr. Callahan's family, decided to discharge her home on hospice and palliative care, in keeping with her advanced directives.

The palliative care physician made a home visit to admit Dr. Callahan to their service and to evaluate her for hospice care. During her intake assessment of Dr. Callahan, the physician asked Dr. Callahan about her illness journey, about her last hospitalization, the pain she has endured, the limitations on her quality of life. Although she was able to respond to many of the questions, it was evident that Dr. Callahan was still confused: she didn't remember that she was just in the hospital but agreed it had been an ordeal; she was surprised that she had a gastric feeding tube (something she'd had for months prior to this last surgery), and she didn't readily recognize her friend who had been involved in her care. Still, Dr. Callahan's responses were mostly consistent with prior conversations and her advanced directives until the last question. When the palliative care physician asked Dr. Callahan what she wanted to have happen if her heart should stop, Dr. Callahan said, "Well you better get it started again." The physician asked if she wanted cardiopulmonary resuscitation (CPR) and go back to the hospital. Dr. Callahan said yes to the CPR but not to the hospitalization.

The physician thanked Dr. Callahan for her time and then asked to speak to the family in the other room. In that conversation, the physician noted that Dr. Callahan was still experiencing delirium from her hospitalization and therefore lacked decisional capacity. She also noted Dr. Callahan's statement that she would want her heart started again if it stopped but that she didn't want to go back to the hospital indicated that she could not fully appreciate the question. Therefore, she continued, it was necessary to look to a time when she had the capacity to determine what should be done going forward—specifically, what Dr. Callahan's code status should be. She pulled out a copy of Dr. Callahan's advanced directives with her additional instructions and said that this statement would provide the guidance needed to make this decision. Based on her advanced directives, Dr. Callahan was made a DNR/DNI and admitted to hospice. The family concurred with that decision and expressed relief that her single statement, expressed during a period of delirium, did not override Dr. Callahan's clear and consistent statement of her advanced directives.

It is important to note that the palliative care physician had been involved in Dr. Callahan's care for several months and had spent time discussing her advanced directives during that period. So, this decision was based on a broader understanding of Dr. Callahan's situation and her expressed preferences than a single conversation. Dr. Callahan died peacefully with family at her side 3 weeks after returning home.

Was it wrong for the palliative care physician to write the DNR/DNI orders? Was Dr. Callahan's statement that she wanted her heart started again an indication that she had changed her mind about her code status? This is where the gnarly part comes in. While we both agree with the physician's decision, we don't pretend to mean that it was the singular right decision to make in that instance. We believe that it was based on careful consideration of Dr. Callahan's situation over the period of her life and her clear and consistent statement of her preferences. Does this mean that we should never listen to the expressed preferences of someone who is experiencing delirium or dementia? No. It means these are complex decisions that require us to delve into the complexity, to try to understand what this older adult might want in this situation. It means that our advanced directives, no matter how clear, will never be able to anticipate every possible situation. Clinicians put this belief into practice by following the standards of person-centered care, by having conversations (repeatedly and over time as their situation changes) with older adults about their preferences. Family members can do the same by avoiding a commitment to a single, fixed rule—like "always keep Mum safe!" or "we want you to try everything possible to save our Dad!"—when involved in making medical and caregiving decisions.

Discussion and Reflection Questions

1. The chapter highlights Dr. Callahan's method of using a table to weigh options for her end-of-life care. How can this approach be adapted and utilized by healthcare teams and families to facilitate more person-centered decisions, especially when persons have difficulty communicating their preferences?
2. What is a hypothetical or real-life scenario where you might encounter a conflict between ensuring a person's safety and respecting their desire for a particular quality of life. Can Dr. Callahan's method be adapted to help make decisions in this case?
3. Advance directives are essential tools for documenting and communicating person preferences. However, it is possible for a person's wishes to change over time. How can healthcare providers ensure that advance directives remain relevant and truly reflect a person's current values, and what role do ongoing conversations play in this process?
4. We have introduced the concepts of "daily decision-making" and observing "patterns of life" as ways to maintain quality of life even when major medical decisions are not being made. How does understanding a person's daily habits and values, even if they cannot communicate, can inform care plans and contribute to their overall well-being and dignity? How can a whole care team ensure that they all share this understanding?

References

Baumrucker SJ, Sheldon JE, Stolick M, Morris GM, Vandekieft G, Harrington D (2008) The ethical concept of 'best interest. Am J Hosp Palliat Care 25(1):56–62

Diekema DS (2011) Revisiting the best interest standard: uses and misuses. J Clin Ethics 22(2):128–133

Kopelman LM (1997) The best-interests standard as threshold, ideal, and standard of reasonableness. J Med Philos 22(3):271–289

Lahey T, Elwyn G (2020) Sliding scale shared decision making for patients with reduced capacity. AMA J Ethics 22(5):E358–E364. https://doi.org/10.1001/amajethics.2020.358

Mellgard G, Gligorov N (2022) Complexity, not severity: reinterpreting the sliding scale of capacity. Camb Q Healthc Ethics 31(4):506–517. https://doi.org/10.1017/S0963180122000111

Menne HL, Whitlatch CJ (2007) Decision-making involvement of individuals with dementia. Gerontologist 47(6):810–819. https://doi.org/10.1093/geront/47.6.810

Miller LM, Whitlatch CJ, Lyons KS (2016) Shared decision-making in dementia: a review of patient and family carer involvement. Dementia 15(5):1141–1157. https://doi.org/10.1177/1471301214555542. Epub 2014 Nov 3

Sawyer KN, Camp-Rogers TR, Kotini-Shah P, Del Rios M, Gossip MR, Moitra VK, Haywood KL et al (2020) Sudden cardiac arrest survivorship: a scientific statement from the American Heart Association. Circulation 141(12):e654–e685

Long-Term Care Facilities and the Staff's Perspective

4

4.1 Case Illustration

Bernita Samuelson is an 87-year-old woman living in an assisted living facility (ALF) who has mobility impairment and is at risk for falls. While she is willing to use her walker when she is ambulating in the ALF, she refuses when she goes on outings because she does not want people to think she is old! Facility staff are concerned that she will fall on an outing and insist she use her walker; if she refuses, she will not be allowed to go.

Bernita has a sister, Julie, who is slightly younger than Bernita, at age 82. She has less severe mobility impairments than Bernita but has a chronic, nonhealing wound of her lower left leg that requires her to have a home health nurse visit two to three times each week to manage the wound. The nurse frequently encourages Julie to consider a move to the ALF to be with Bernita. They try to convince her that she will have more socialization. However, Julie prefers to remain in the childhood home that she and Bernita inherited when their parents died two decades ago and which soon after became Julie's primary residence. Living in this home helps Julie feel connected to her family. Like Bernita, she does not want people to think she is old—so she rarely leaves the house. She has food delivered and hires a cleaning service to help maintain the family home—her home. When she visits Bernita, the ALF staff tell her how much it would mean to Bernita if Julie moved there. Nevertheless, Julie insists on remaining in her home.

4.2 Chapter Outline

Long-term care (LTC) staff are faced with dilemmas that pit concerns about safety against a person's autonomy and quality of life almost every day and with nearly every resident—the person living with diabetes who loves ice cream and wants to eat it every day, the older adult at high risk of falling who refuses to use a walker,

T. A. Harvath, M. Fedyk, *What If Maslow Was Wrong?*, https://doi.org/10.1007/978-3-032-14249-8_4

the older gentleman who is on several opioid medications for severe arthritis pain who enjoys a glass of scotch every evening. These dilemmas are routine in nursing homes.

Because of this, LTC staff have developed strategies for working with these dilemmas. We stress the importance of the phrase "working with"—these are just the default strategies that LTC staff have. These strategies often reflect a bias toward safety and minimizing risk. They are neither the best nor only solutions to the dilemmas. In fact, many of the LTC staff we have worked with in our careers would be quite happy to have better strategies than the defaults; they would be excited to develop "improved" strategies with residents and their caregivers because they can see the impact of safety (or the illusion of safety as we have noted before) on quality of life for the residents. So, we will offer some suggestions about some "improved" strategies in both this and subsequent chapters.

The main purpose of this chapter is to introduce some of the regulatory guidance that holds LTC staff accountable when managing resident preferences that involve risk. We hope therefore that this chapter helps residents and families develop deeper insight into how LTC staff think about older adults like Julie and Bernita. That said, after the tour, we'll offer a suggestion about how LTC staff can more effectively balance safety with quality of life and autonomy—potentially changing how they view older adults like the Samuelson sisters.

As we said in the introduction, many of the topics we touch on in this chapter will be explored more deeply in subsequent chapters. So, please don't worry if we seem to move too quickly when discussing an idea or a rule that seems important—please just keep reading!

4.3 Nursing Homes and the Safety Mandate

In 1987, as part of the Omnibus Budget Reconciliation Act (OBRA), the US Congress passed the Nursing Home Reform Act (Public Law. No. 100-203 1987). This legislation implemented an era of sweeping reform in nursing homes through the creation of a set of national standards for care, a formal quality assurance process, and a system for enforcement of these new standards (Weiner et al. 2007). This reform was a response to widespread concerns about the poor quality of care in nursing homes.

These reforms are the foundation of the operational practices of most nursing homes. In 2007, Weiner, Freiman, and Samuelson published a report analyzing the impact of the OBRA 1987 regulations on the quality of nursing home care. This report points out that a major focus of long-term care regulation is on resident health and safety, with a specific focus on markers of poor care quality—e.g., pressure ulcers and malnutrition. The authors also note that very little data is available that assesses the quality of life for nursing home residents, in part, because these include "intangible factors, such as autonomy, individuality, comfort, meaningful activity and relationships, a sense of security, and spiritual well-being" (pg. 9). In other words, nursing homes were effectively mandated by the 1987 OBRA to prioritize measuring and monitoring safety over measuring and monitoring quality of life.

This is an important finding because a growing body of research demonstrates the importance of resident autonomy to their quality of life (Bhattacharyya et al. 2021; McCabe et al. 2021; Moilanen et al. 2021). A recent report by the National Academies (2022) presents a comprehensive review of nursing home quality and provides recommendations that emphasize the importance of resident autonomy and quality of life, in addition to safety and care quality. The first goal that this review identified was "Deliver Comprehensive, person-centered, equitable care that ensures the health, quality of life, and safety of nursing home residents; promotes resident autonomy and manages risks" (National Academies 2022, pg. 5).

This goal is significant because it states clearly that it is not enough to provide care that meets residents' basic needs and does not cause harm. Instead, long-term care residents have a right to expect that the care they receive will enhance their quality of life and respect their autonomy. Still, these calls for change have not produced the intended effect—for instance, there is still a bias toward safety in the language of regulatory documents and national reports of nursing home quality. A basic word search of some of the most important regulatory documents demonstrates a disproportionate emphasis on safety compared to quality of life and autonomy (Table 4.1).

What the National Academies' report and other regulatory documents fail to address is how to manage the dynamic tension that exists when resident autonomy and expressed preferences raise concerns for their safety and the safety of others in the building. Instead, they provide guidance that encourages the nursing home staff to try multiple approaches to gain the resident's cooperation:

> In situations where a resident's choice to decline care or treatment (e.g., due to preferences, maintain autonomy, etc.) poses a risk to the resident's health or safety, the comprehensive care plan must identify the care or service being declined, the risk the declination poses to the resident, and efforts by the interdisciplinary team to educate the resident and the representative, as appropriate. (CMS State Operations Manual, Appendix PP, pp. 240)

This language requires the members of the interdisciplinary team to try to persuade (through education) the resident to comply with the care or treatment. There is also language that runs through these regulatory documents that provides the caveat that residents' preferences can be curtailed if they pose a risk for the resident or other people (i.e., other residents, visitors, and staff). Implicit in this language is that safety trumps resident autonomy and quality of life—if only because, when push

Table 4.1 Frequency of key concepts cited in nursing home regulations and major reports

Report/document	Safety	Quality of life	Autonomy
Institute of Medicine (1986)	80	107	5
CMS State Operations Manual, Appendix PP (2023)	369	101	21
CSC 42 CFR 483 (2023)	119	8	1
National Academies (2022)	236	184	37
Total	**804**	**400**	**64**

comes to shove, (metaphorically speaking) regulatory agencies and the courts will care about safety more than they will care about autonomy.

These observations might help explain the ALF staff's stance toward Julie and Bernita. It is not that the staff were unaware of the importance of not being perceived as old to Bernita or the importance of living in the family home to Julie. Some of the regulatory guidance tells them to focus on these important aspects of the Samuelson sister's lives. However, safety matters most. As a result, operationally, the staff of long-term care facilities will usually try to persuade residents and their families to make decisions that align with these underlying concerns for safety.

4.4 Conflated Meanings of Safety

Back in Chap. 2, we introduced you to four common ways that "safety" is defined when providing care to older adults. There is *safety as error reduction*, *safety as liability reduction*, *safety as taking away the freedom to make choices*, and *safety as physical harm reduction*. The biggest idea in that chapter is that if you keep these meanings of "safety" separate, you can then look at different environments as different "safety-generating social systems" that will produce differing amounts of these four different kinds of safety. By "adding up" the safety produced in different environments, we might discover that Julie is safer at home than moving in with her sister.

Unfortunately, when safety is discussed by national regulatory bodies and oversight agencies, the different meanings of "safety" are run together, for example, an entire chapter in the recent National Academies' report (2022) was devoted to "ensuring the safety of nursing home residents" (pp. 303–356). In this report, the term "safety" is frequently used to mean both error and physical harm reduction. The report also defines medication safety as ensuring that residents receive the right medication in the right dose at the right time; note that this particular definition of safety is very strongly biased against the view that someone like Julie is safe at home—as every nurse knows, making sure a person, no matter how old or young they are, always takes the right medicine at the right time and in the right way at home is difficult. Our point is that it is too easy to use the concept of medical safety as a reason to conclude that someone like Julie is not safe living in her home—if, that is, there are medications that she should be taking.

The authors of the National Academies' report also cite a report from the Office of the Inspector General (2014) that documented that over half of the harms experienced by nursing home residents are "preventable," including falls or omission of care. However, labeling these harms as preventable—and thereby linking them to the concept of safety as error reduction—obscures the complexity that belies this issue. Interventions that may reduce falls can impinge on a resident's movements. Omissions of care may reflect honoring a resident's right to refuse care or treatment. Importantly, the report acknowledges that "nursing homes must balance safety with residents' preferences for autonomy and quality of life" (National Academies 2022, pg. 303). Unfortunately, they provide little guidance in how to achieve that balance—and much of the language is consistent with the idea often borrowed from

Maslow, that safety must be "maximized" first, rather than one of the several distinct outcomes that must be balanced when making impossible choices.

Safety as error reduction is probably the easiest kind of safety to measure. As a result, well-intentioned efforts to "protect" residents inspired by reports like the National Academies document can lead to situations in which this becomes the only meaning of safety (and consequently the only measures of care quality) that matters—which further complicates efforts to balance safety with quality of life and autonomy—for example, nursing homes have dramatically increased the use of tab or bed alarm over the last 25 years. These alarms are devices attached either to the resident or their bed so that staff are alerted when the resident tries to get up unassisted (Crogan and Dupler 2014). These alarms are often viewed as important "safeguards" that are implemented to protect unrestrained residents from falling. However, there is no strong evidence to suggest that tab alarms *prevent* residents from falling (Anderson et al. 2012; Chan et al. 2021; Crogan and Dupler 2014). Indeed, one study showed a reduction in falls after the alarms were removed (Crogan and Dupler 2014). Further, some evidence suggests the alarms can add to the environmental noise pollution causing stress for residents and staff alike (Oh-Park et al. 2021). However, because the alarms provide a mechanism to continuously monitor residents, they generate an illusion of safety. Anyone who wants to know whether residents were safe can just look at the telemetry data generated by these alarms. But as we've shown, there are at least four other kinds of safety that could matter—Julie might have less risk of injury from fall if she moves in with Bernita, but this does not mean that, considering all the meanings of "safety," Julie would be safer living in a nursing home with Bernita.

4.5 Resident Autonomy and Risk

The assumption that it is possible to protect nursing home residents from harm is inherent in policy language that describes falls and other adverse events as "preventable" (National Academies 2022). This language is important because it presumes that the facility staff could have done something to avoid these adverse events. While that may be true in some situations, it is often more complicated, for example, facilities are required to refrain from using physical restraints but can be faulted when a resident, who is unsteady, falls. Similarly, a facility can be cited for nutritional deficits when a resident is refusing to eat. These situations put the staff in a difficult position of trying to provide care that the resident does not want. Language in several regulatory documents (see, for example, CMS State Operations Manual, Appendix PP 2023) instructs nursing home personnel to "educate" the resident if their choice poses risks for the resident and requires that staff document the alternative treatments offered. This language pushes staff to override resident's preferences to avoid raising concerns with surveyors. It also implies that a resident's choice is an uninformed choice and if we just educate them they will make a "better" choice.

Pioneer Network, an organization devoted to changing the culture of aging to become more person-centered, recognizes that risk is an inherent part of life (Vision,

Mission, & Values 2016). This is an important ethical idea. For older adults, including older adults in nursing homes, activities that may carry risk can often contribute to quality of life or reflect the resident's expression of autonomy. When faced with a situation where the expressed preferences of nursing home residents involve some perceived risk, we often ignore, disregard, or minimize their stated preferences and the impact on their quality of life. The rationale is based on the "promotion of safety" or on the interpretation of state and federal regulations. However, it is important to emphasize that while protecting vulnerable nursing home residents is important, it is also important to recognize the trade-offs that come with "protective" measures. It is essential that the risks to resident quality of life and autonomy that come with attempts to keep nursing home residents "safe" are not ignored. (We'll explore how to navigate some of these trade-offs in the next four chapters.)

It is also important to mention that clinical research does not decisively favor promoting safety as error reduction above all other considerations. For example, a recent paper reveals that restricting resident autonomy in nursing homes is associated with poorer health outcomes (Moilanen et al. 2021). What's more, in their critical review of literature on the effects of autonomy (or lack thereof) on the health and well-being of nursing home residents, the same researchers found in study after study that promoting autonomy was correlated with improved subjective health, better coping strategies, positive mental health, and an enhanced sense of self-worth and dignity (Moilanen et al. 2021).

4.6 Proposed Framework: The Three-Legged Stool

So, how can the staff of nursing homes address some of the biases and patterns that we've examined? We suggest that they use a mental model that takes the idea that safety should be balanced with autonomy and quality of life very, well, *literally*. We suggest that when providing care to residents or people like Bernita or Julie, staff should form a mental model of a wobbly stool with three legs—each leg standing for safety, autonomy, and quality of life. The wobble is important: the stool is never going to be perfectly balanced. It will be tipsy. Still, unless one of the legs is disproportionately longer or shorter than the other two, a three-legged stool will balance and not topple over. The point is just to make sure the stool isn't going to fall over if anyone sits on it. What will make the stool topple? If, for example, there is way too much emphasis on safety, that leg will be longer than the legs for autonomy and quality of life, and the chair will be at risk for tipping.

When making any decision that impacts a resident or even when simply offering advice, we invite LTC staff to engage in a moment of critical reflection and ask: Does this increase or decrease the amount of wobble in the stool? If it decreases the wobble, then the decision is probably a good decision to make—we have some balance between safety, autonomy, and quality of life. It if increases the wobble, then maybe alternatives should be searched for—or attention should be put toward further actions or interventions that ameliorate the additional wobble. Each resident's stool will wobble in a different way—and that of course is perfectly fine—because that is a sign that the resident is being treated as a unique individual with their own personal values.

In Bernita's situation, it is important to recognize that Bernita's preference is based on her sense of dignity; attributing her desire to eschew her walker as denial of risk, vanity, or poor judgment fails to recognize that she is making a choice that makes sense to her, reflects her values, and is important to her. Her choices help ensure that the autonomy and quality of life legs of her stool do not become too short.

We believe this way of balancing safety with autonomy and quality of life could invite a more critical analysis of the risks that Bernita faces in participating in the outings without her walker and how to ameliorate those risks. How big a risk for falling does Ms. Samuelson really have? Are there any resources (e.g., volunteers, family members) who could help to reduce that risk by walking closely with Ms. Samuelson? Does the outing present specific risks (e.g., uneven surfaces) that might be important to consider? Is Ms. Samuelson or her family willing to assume some risk (e.g., sign waivers) so that quality of life can be enhanced? What are the risks involved in Ms. Samuelson being left out of outings (e.g., loneliness and social isolation)? In short, are their steps that can be taken to ensure that Bernita's stool doesn't get too wobbly?

4.7 Conclusion

Ultimately, Julie did decide to move in with Bernita. But not because she believed she would be safer joining her sister in the nursing home. Instead, her perceptions shifted after several months of taking a taxi across town to visit Bernita in her apartment at the nursing home. Julie realized that Bernita, being the only member of her family still alive, was a more important source of connection with her family than the house. In other words, Julie realized that her quality of life would be improved by spending more time with her sister. Julie was also happy to join Bernita on the outings planned by the nursing home, which decreased the stress that the nursing home staff felt—because Julie helped Bernita maintain her balance while also maintaining her dignity. This, thankfully, is a story that ends well.

It also reveals something important. If the nursing home staff had not engaged with Bernita and Julie from only a perspective of safety, then it might have been easier to find a solution that decreased the wobble in both Julie's and Bernita's stool. In fact, too much focus on safety can sometimes backfire—causing permanent reductions in safety, autonomy, or quality of life. We will examine exactly this paradox later in Chap. 6. In the meantime, we want to go deeper into a case that has some features in common with the case of the Samuelson sisters, one that helps use clarify the important difference between independence and autonomy.

Discussion and Reflection Questions

1. The chapter introduces the "three-legged stool" framework, emphasizing that safety, autonomy, and quality of life must be balanced, not prioritized. How does

this concept challenge traditional approaches to resident care, particularly in nursing homes?

2. We have discussed how different meanings of "safety" (error reduction, liability reduction, freedom reduction, physical harm reduction) are often conflated in regulatory documents. How might distinguishing between these types of safety change how healthcare LTC staff assess and manage risk for older adults?
3. The chapter suggests that regulatory documents often implicitly prioritize safety, even when acknowledging the importance of autonomy and quality of life. How might this regulatory environment influence the decisions and practices of nursing home staff, and what are the potential consequences for residents?
4. The Pioneer Network's philosophy, recognizing risk as inherent in life, is an important ethical idea. How can healthcare LTC staff integrate this perspective into their care plans while still ensuring responsible and ethical care for older adults?

References

Anderson O, Boshier PR, Hanna GB (2012) Interventions designed to prevent healthcare bed-related injuries in patients. Cochrane Database Syst Rev 1(1):CD008931. PMID: 22258994; PMCID: PMC11569887. https://doi.org/10.1002/14651858.CD008931 .pub3

Bhattacharyya KK, Molinari V, Hyer K (2021) Self-reported satisfaction of older adult residents in nursing homes: development of a conceptual framework. Gerontologist 62(8):e442–e456

Chan DKY, Chan LKM, Kuang YM, Celler B (2021) Digital care technologies in people with dementia living in long-term facilities to prevent falls and manage behavioural and psychological symptoms of dementia: a systematic review. Eur J Aging 19:309–323

CMS State Operations Manual, Appendix PP – Guidance to surveyors for long-term care facilities (2023) https://www.cms.gov/medicare/provider-enrollment-and-certification/guidanceforlawsandregulations/downloads/appendix-pp-state-operations-manual.pdf

Crogan NL, Dupler AE (2014) Quality improvement in nursing homes: testing an alarm elimination program. J Nurs Care Qual 29(1):60–65

Institute of Medicine (1986) Improving the quality of care in nursing homes. National Academy Press, Washington, DC. https://doi.org/10.17226/646

McCabe M, Byers J, Busija L, Mellor D, Bennett M, Beattie E (2021) How important are choice, autonomy, and relationships in predicting the quality of life of nursing home residents? J Appl Gerontol 40(12):1743–1750. Epub 2021 Jan 6. PMID: 33402014. https://doi.org/10.1177/0733464820983972

Moilanen T, Kangasniemi M, Papinaho O, Mynttinen M, Siipi H, Souminen S, Suhonen R (2021) Older people's perceived autonomy in residential care: an integrative review. Nurs Ethics 28(3):414–434

National Academies of Sciences, Engineering, and Medicine (2022) The national imperative to improve nursing home quality: honoring our commitment to residents, families, and staff. The National Academies Press, Washington, DC. https://doi.org/10.17226/26526

Oh-Park M, Doan T, Dohle C, Vermiglio-Kohn V, Abdou A (2021) Technology utilization in fall prevention. Am J Phys Med Rehabil 100(1):92–99

Omnibus Budget Reconciliation Act of 1987, Public Law. No. 100-203 (1987)

U.S. Department of Health and Human Services, Office of the Inspector General (2014) Adverse events in skilled nursing facilities: national incidence among Medicare beneficiaries. Office of Evaluation and Inspections, Washington, DC. OEI-06-11-00370

Vision, Mission & Values (2016) Pioneer Network. October 5, 2016. https://www.pioneernetwork.org/about-us/mission-vision-values/

Weiner JM, Freiman MP, Samuelson D (2007) Nursing home care quality: twenty years after the Omnibus Budget Reconciliation Act of 1987. Kaiser Family Foundation

Independence Versus Autonomy

5

5.1 Case Illustration

Michael Wong is a 72-year-old man who is quadriplegic because of his multiple sclerosis. Mr. Wong is a resident in a Veterans Administration nursing home where he is completely dependent on others for most of his activities of daily living (ADLs). Mr. Wong uses an electric wheelchair with proportional chin control for his mobility. With that setup, he can propel himself independently around environments that are wheelchair accessible. He requires the assistance of two certified nursing assistants (CNAs) for his bathing, dressing, toileting, and transfers. He needs to be fed but can drink through a straw if his cup is placed in a cupholder on the wheelchair tray.

Mr. Wong enjoys working with students. They are often surprised to hear him describe himself as 100% independent. He goes on to explain, "If I want to have pizza, I get someone to order it for me. If I want to go to the mall, I get someone to schedule the wheelchair van."

Mr. Wong lives next door to Mr. Gregory, a 93-year-old man with chronic severe osteoarthritis that also creates mobility challenges for him. When Mr. Wong is waiting in the hallway, he and Mr. Gregory will sometimes chat about the different ways in which they feel that they have preserved their independence. They often find themselves agreeing about the value of finding ways of continuing activities that express their deepest values.

5.2 Chapter Outline

In this chapter, we turn to a topic that is central to the ethics of elderly care. We've spent a lot of time now exploring how to separate safety from autonomy and quality of life. But on the other side of autonomy is the concept of independence, and, as we

T. A. Harvath, M. Fedyk, *What If Maslow Was Wrong?*,
https://doi.org/10.1007/978-3-032-14249-8_5

will use the case example of Mr. Wong to illustrate, getting to a deeper understanding of the distinction between independence and autonomy can help address some of the impossible choices related to autonomy.

5.3 Autonomy and Independence

So, let us start with the distinction. Mr. Wong is probably referring to his autonomy when he says he is 100% independent. This conflation is understandable, because these terms are often used interchangeably in healthcare. But the terms "autonomy" and "independence" express very different concepts, especially when discussing the ethics of caring of older adults. In fact, the two terms probably should always be kept separate, no matter the context. Here is why: no one can live independently of the efforts of any other person. The division of labor—how we use our unique talents and abilities to help others while benefiting from their unique talents and abilities—ensures that, at a very deep level, every living person is dependent on countless other people, who are themselves just as dependent on another group of people, and so on. In short, we are all share a need for interdependence: no one enjoys even the most minimal levels of food, shelter, or necessities (remember Maslow!) without participating in relationships of mutual dependence. No one is 100% independent. We all need other people to survive.

Autonomy has much less to do with survival and cooperation. Instead, it is easiest to understand autonomy as a concept that is about values or, more specifically, one person's values. We suggest that it is most helpful to think of autonomy as a "dial" that measures the congruence between a person's values and how they live their life. The more congruence there is between their day-to-day world and their values, the more autonomy the person has, and the less congruence between a person's values and their day-to-day life, the less autonomy they have.

Clinicians have invented several popular conceptual frameworks that are different versions of the "dial" of autonomy. We've already discussed one of the most common: the ethical framework that is called "person-centered care." This is an attempt to ensure that no person's autonomy dial falls too low: all the interventions that a care team makes on behalf of an older adult should reflect—to the degree possible—choices that the person makes. This isn't because choosing between different options for care is what matters. Indeed, the most important ethical component of person-centered care is the idea that choices are how a person makes their values known to the care team—these choices should be the source of congruence between the person's values and how they are treated.

At this point, ethics discussions usually turn to three ideas about how to ensure that a person's choices really do further their autonomy. These are the concepts of informed decision-making (Does a person know enough about the medical facts of their situation to integrate their values and their choices?), capacity (Is the person alert and aware enough to make decisions?), and voluntariness (Is the person making choices in a situation in which nothing is interfering with the ability of their values to shape their choices? Are they free of manipulation or coercion?). But instead, we want to shift focus to some less abstract but equally important issues that arise when thinking about the autonomy of older adults—because this gets us back to the difference between autonomy and independence.

As we age, we often become less independent. We need more help from friends, family, and strangers to have either our highest values realized or, increasingly, our most basic needs met. Here, we encounter a cornerstone in the care of older adults: the focus on maintaining, promoting, and restoring functional capacities impacted by aging, illness, or even just bad luck—and in so doing, helping them as much as possible to get back to less dependence and more independence. Nurses and doctors have a term for this: they talk about a person's function—their ability to perform their instrumental activities of daily living (IADLs) (e.g., shopping, transportation, etc.) and their activities of daily living (ADLs) (e.g., bathing, dressing, etc.). Older adults who can perform their ADLs without assistance are often referred to as "independent" in those activities. If, however, an older adult needs the assistance of another person to perform their ADLs, they are referred to as "dependent" in those activities. A goal of care may be to "promote independence" in those activities so that the older person can perform those activities without assistance—and this goal can be an expression of a person's autonomy if it is something that they choose because it brings congruence between their values and how they are living. This is how autonomy and independence can overlap; it explains how the terms "autonomy" and "independence" can become interchangeable.

But what if promoting independence in ADLs is not congruent with an older adults' values? Some older adults find it taxing or painful to do their own ADLs. Instead, they may prefer to receive assistance from others. When an older adult *directs* another person in the performance of those ADLs, they are still considered "autonomous" in their ADLs even while dependent on others to carry out the activities—because, again, their choices are shaping their situation in ways that allows the choices to be a means by which congruence between the older person's values and their lived reality is maintained.

Unfortunately, we often neglect to make or value that important distinction when planning care for older adults. Remember that Mr. Gregory, who we introduced you to above, has severe osteoarthritis that limits how easy it is for him to move his arms and legs. As a result, walking with a walker or trying to propel his wheelchair by himself caused great pain for him in his hips and shoulders. It was not unusual for him to sit in his wheelchair outside his room and flag down a passing staff member to ask to be pushed to the community room, as he deeply valued connecting with other people. His requests for assistance were often met with an encouragement to try to get there on his own. It is not that the staff weren't interested in helping Mr. Gregory. The reason is that his care plan had a goal of independent wheelchair mobility; no one had thought to ask whether Mr. Gregory valued more than just physical mobility. As a result, the interventions described in his care plan instructed staff to encourage him to get himself to the community room under his own efforts. If, on the other hand, Mr. Gregory's care plan had a goal of social connection, the interventions would likely be very different.

When discussing Mr. Gregory's case with students, one student pointed out that she considers herself to be "functionally independent" in her transportation even though she rides the bus to work and to school. She noted that she doesn't drive the bus but knows how to access it to get around town. She went on to suggest that when Mr. Gregory was flagging down staff to get a push, he was simply "hailing a cab," using the transportation supports available to him in the facility. It is important to note that when staff would give Mr. Gregory a ride, he often regaled them with a story, not keeping them too long from their work but just enough to get a quick interaction. If we understand that Mr. Gregory had the goals of getting to the community room with as little pain as possible and to interact with staff and other veterans for a brief period, we understand better how his values relate to his requests for assistance.

Too often in long-term care we interpret an older person's request for help as an inappropriate desire for attention or perhaps even laziness in the face of physical difficulties. We assume that they want what we think we would want if we were in their position—to get around by one's own means. If, instead, we understood the meaning of the request from the perspective of autonomy and valued efforts to express autonomy, we might better enact person-centered or person-directed care. A simple test of whether a goal in a plan of care for an older adult respects their autonomy is put it in first-person language. Can you imagine that Mr. Gregory would say, "If I ask you to push me to the community room, please encourage me to do it by myself." That language may make sense for someone who is rehabilitating from a knee replacement, and their goal is to return home. Given what we know about Mr. Gregory, does the language make sense for him?

5.4 Person-Centered Care, Autonomy, and Choice

Generally speaking, when we talk about person-centered care, we think of honoring an older adult's choices. "Does Mr. Gregory want to go to bingo this afternoon?" "Does Mr. Wong know about the new pizza place that opened up nearby?" "Do you think that Mr. Gregory and Mr. Wong might enjoy playing scrabble together?" Each of these questions has a particular goal in mind: adding more pleasure and meaning to the lives of older adults. Because of that, each question presupposes a specific way of thinking about what values are: values *as* desires. The thinking here is that by asking these questions of Mr. Wong and Mr. Gregory we discover their desires and we can then support their autonomy by taking actions that satisfy these desires. Going further, we can increase the autonomy of Mr. Gregory and Mr. Wong by asking them questions that probe for any desires that they might not have expressed yet. Maybe Mr. Wong likes Chinese food just as much as Mr. Gregory likes pizza; maybe Mr. Gregory would enjoy speaking to new residents of an assisted living facility.

However, there is another way of thinking about values that, in the history of ethics, has a deeper connection with autonomy. This is the idea that a person's values are the principles that they would choose over everything else. Ethicists usually link this idea to Kant, as he was one of the first thinkers to explore how this idea can unlock an even more powerful concept of autonomy. Thankfully, we don't need to engage with Kant here—as the idea that principles are different from desires is enough to say some useful things about how to explore deeper ways of supporting Mr. Wong or Mr. Gregory's autonomy.

We slipped the idea of congruence between a person's values and their situation into our discussion because it helps us get to a set of deeper ideas that, once understood, can help persons, families, and providers better navigate the balancing act involved in protecting an older adult's autonomy in the face of decreases in functional independence. Specifically, the idea that autonomy is obtained—even if imperfectly—through congruence between a person's values and their living situation helps us get a better handle on the kinds of questions and conversations that persons, providers, and families can have when thinking about the care of older adults.

Let's step back, then, and reflect a bit more on what it means for there to be congruence between a person's values and their lived experience. It certainly is the case that if some of our more important desires are routinely filled, this counts as an important amount of congruence. But examining a person's desires is not the only way to figure out what they value. Why? Well, it is easy for our desires to come into conflict, either with themselves, with other beliefs, or with plans, or as often happens in the care of older adults, an older person's desires might come into conflict with the desires of their caregivers or family members or other residents if they live in a congregate care environment. Furthermore, desires, when satisfied, tend to go away—but does that mean that the person no longer values what they (at least for the moment) no longer desire? Desires can be disorganized, transient, and even irrational. Trying to meet the desires of every single older adult, especially every older adult in long-term care, would not only be impossible but would also result in utter chaos and be a nightmare for all involved. Thus, it is perhaps better to look for something deeper than desires.

All the same, we have both participated in many family conferences in which the meeting begins with someone saying "Ok—we are here to figure out what everyone wants, and then we'll help you form a plan that helps everyone achieve those goals." Similarly, many goals of care interviews with persons begin with the provider assuming, reasonably enough, that goals that are linked to desires are the only goals worth talking about. These interviews might start "Mr. Wong, we're here to help figure out what goals you have for your care. Can you tell me some of your most important wishes for your care?" Desires become the focuses of providers and caregivers because they are easy for a person to talk about.

Getting at the principles that underlie values and desires can be more difficult to ascertain. We want therefore to offer some suggestions about how to talk about principles in a way that, while not quite as easy as talking about desires (i.e., wants, wishes, goals), unlocks the ability to explore deeper levels of value congruence and thus even more powerful forms of autonomy.

5.5 Talking About Principles

So let us go back to the scenario in which Mr. Gregory's care team is talking to him to develop a care plan. What kinds of questions could they ask that would help them uncover principles—rather than desires—that Mr. Gregory holds, and which would, if used as the basis of his care plan, provide a deeper expression of Mr. Gregory's autonomy? The answer to this question is that the care team should ask about values that "transcend" the local circumstances of care, for example, rather than asking what Mr. Gregory wants given that he is livening in an assisted living facility, ask him about what patterns in his life have been persisted longest and with which Mr. Gregory identifies.

We introduced you to the idea of patterns of life back in Chap. 3. But that discussion was relatively brief, and we are not using the concept in a distinction that is quite so abstract. So let us spend a bit more time investigating Mr. Gregory's personal history to explore how to make his patterns of life more concrete. We can tell you now that Mr. Gregory has a refined and sophisticated sense of sartorial style, one of the best we've ever seen in a person. For most of his life, he wore tailored trousers and shirts, nicely made leather shoes, and a selection of custom-made gentleman's hats. In family photos, Mr. Gregory always stands out for how put together he looks, and he keeps part of his closet in the nursing home reserved for some of his "greatest hits"—outfits that no longer fit him, with which he clearly still identifies—you never know when the occasion might arise where that outfit would be just the right thing! Mr. Gregory's sense of style is one of the "principles" of his life. It is a "pattern" that runs through his whole life.

But now, living in the VA nursing home, with his severe osteoarthritis, Mr. Gregory has lost the ability to dress himself with minimal effort. In fact, it usually takes him over an hour of deliberate and painful work to dress himself—and what's worse, the clothes that he ends up putting on do not always match. His care team is concerned, but they are also most focused on the pain that Mr. Gregory experiences and the amount of time it takes him to get ready. This is the point where "talking about principles rather than desires" makes a difference.

If Mr. Gregory's care team focuses on immediate desires—like seeing his friends for breakfast or, even more basically, avoiding pain—they may focus their questions on matters of the type of assistance he needs. Would Mr. Gregory like some help picking out his clothes and getting dressed? With this assistance, he would have less pain and more social connection. After all, this is the same man who "hails" nursing home staff from his wheelchair to help him get around—wouldn't he want the same help getting dressed? And these are not inappropriate ways to provide care to Mr. Gregory. It is when we lose sight of Mr. Gregory because we have now set a new pattern into place, one that persists every day over time.

But if Mr. Gregory's care team focuses on "principles"—again, decades-long patterns that have persisted across deep changes in personal situation—then the considerations are different. The key idea here is that these principles have literally shaped Mr. Gregory into who he is: his identity as a person is a by-product of thousands and thousands of past choices that made him into who he is. More than that, they made who he is congruent with his own values. He used his autonomy to shape himself. From this perspective, Mr. Gregory's efforts to dress himself, even if they are slow and not always sartorially well-composed, reflect some of his deepest values. He is continuing to exercise his autonomy even if the end product of these expressions of his principles are not what they used to be.

So, the suggestion here is that a care team can learn about a person's principles by asking questions about person's life—exploring habits or practices that have persisted across big changes in a person's life. In Mr. Gregory's case, we can learn that he identifies with his sartorial sense from his stories and his pictures: as we said above, fashion is a pattern that is central to Mr. Gregory's life. His life would have been very different—and it would have had very different meaning for him—if this pattern had not been there. And that insight right there is the key to asking the kinds of questions which help caregivers and providers learn about the relevant patterns: ask—or try to learn—how a person's life would have been very different in its meaning to them if what seems to be a principle of their life had not been present. So, instead of assuming we got it right the first time in deciding that what Mr. Gregory needs is assistance with dressing, what would happen if we asked occasionally "Is today a day you want to mix it up a bit, maybe get a little dressed up, put on a tie?" In doing so, we communicate to Mr. Gregory that we recognize that while pain control is important, so is his self-identity, something that has been shaped over a lifetime of choices. Perhaps Mr. Gregory's life would have been different if he had developed a different wardrobe over the years—perhaps not. But his life would likely have had very different meaning to him—it would have expressed very different principles—if he was not able to express his refined sense of fashion.

5.6 Safety Is Not a First Principle

At this point, we can return to a problem that we talked about in the first chapters—the problem of how to think about safety when considering the care of older adults. One way of summarizing this book's message in a single sentence is safety is not a Kantian principle. No one—or, well, almost no one!—will personally identify with a life lived according to maximum safety. Instead, most of life consists of taking different kinds of risks to realize something that is valuable because it is a principle of a person's life. This could be education (risks: long-term debt, exhaustion, discouragement), marriage (risks: financial instability, incompatible in-laws, long-term care obligations), friendship (risks: emotional betrayal, financial obligations, stress from nonreciprocated caregiving), or any number of the things that most of us pursue as central elements of our lives. By the time an older adult is considering whether to move into an assisted living facility, their life story will reveal the presence of several principles and almost never will safety be among these. Even those situations where the older adult says they are doing it for reasons of safety, there is often another principle-motivated rationale (e.g., my kids keep worrying about me; I don't want to be a burden to my children).

In fact, we can build on this important observation. Recall Maslow's hierarchy: it has five levels, the highest of which refers to self-actualization, which is of course a short hand for the idea that a person can make choices that usually cause their life to be organized around their deepest held principles. We have been arguing in this chapter is that it is easy to forget about the highest levels of Maslow's hierarchy: most institutional models for nursing homes or assisted living facilities, for instance, effectively only prioritize levels 1 and 2 by focusing most time, energy, and money on food, shelter, and safety. Safety might matter because it is necessary for a person like Mr. Gregory to be able to spend time in the morning selecting his outfit for the day, but it does not matter as much or in the same way that Mr. Gregory's sartorial sense matters to him.

Ethicists think that these distinctions are very important—so important that there is standardized vocabulary for talking about this distinction. We want to try to teach you this vocabulary, because we can then use it to summarize the deeper points we are trying to share in this chapter. So, here is the distinction. Goals, projects, desires, habits, and practices—in short, all the sorts of things that a person can imagine either wanting to do or using as the motivation to do something—are called ends. How someone pursues any of their "ends" are the "means."

So far, so good, but here are the complicating factors. Means and ends do not just stand in a one-to-one relationship in anyone's lives: long-term or deeply important ends (marriage, education, living to 100) may only be realized if someone pursues hundreds of more immediate ends (staying fit, learning how to study, watching how much sugar is present in one's diet), and each of these more immediate ends may in turn depend upon hundreds of even more immediate ends. The choices a person makes in their day-to-day life are all choices that happen within the structure—or the fabric—of the complex structure of ends and means. Now, once you can see this structure in a person's life, you can ask one of the most important questions in ethics: what sorts of things the person is pursuing as "ends for their own sake" and what sorts of things are they perusing as "ends for the sake of some other end." Mr. Wong may value working with students because it reminds him of his father, who was a skilled teacher that Mr. Wong greatly admired—if so, then Mr. Wong values working with students because of (the further end of) helping him stay connected with memories of his parents. Alternatively, Mr. Wong may value working with students for no other reason than he finds great value in working with students—in which case, for Mr. Gregory, working with students is an "end for its own sake." There is no further point or purpose, at least for Mr. Gregory, of working with students.

The standardized vocabulary that ethicists use to describe these ideas is that, in a person's life, all the person's ends are either ends in themselves or ends to other ends. The idea here is more important than the vocabulary, however, because if you can ask older adults like Mr. Wong or Mr. Gregory what sorts of things they have always done or would like to keep doing, just "for its own sake and for no other reason," then you have identified some of the principles of their lives. And if you asked either of these men whether they pursued safety for its own sake, then both would tell you "Of course not! What kind of life would that be!?!"

Safety matters—but is matters only to other ends. Safety is not an "end in itself." Indeed, a study assessing how older adults prioritized needs from Maslow's hierarchy (Majercsik 2005) found that older adults valued self-actualization and esteem more highly than safety. Autonomy is being able to live so that one's life, in some way or another, expresses the values that, for a person, are "ends in themselves"—things that are done for their own sake, and which are therefore liable to be the foundation of the person's life patterns. Keeping in mind the difference between independence and autonomy helps us build care plans that preserve autonomy. There is something deeply important about ensuring Mr. Wong can order pizza and Mr. Gregory can dress as he chooses, for as long as it is practical to do so. Focusing too much on safety can lead us to misunderstand the value these things have for these two men.

5.7 Integrating Autonomy into Day-to-Day Care

Let us try to bring that distinction into closer contact with the day-to-day concerns that care staff usually have when working with residents in long-term care facilities. Here is a Table 5.1 that contrasts a "safety-focused" with an "autonomy-focused" approach.

A long-term care facility that focuses only on the safety column will ultimately be organized around custodial care that has all the objective features of a very safe place to live. But a long-term care facility that discovers how to balance concerns

Table 5.1 Safety-focused versus autonomy-focused care planning

	Safety-focused	Autonomy-focused
Food	Are residents getting sufficient calories? Is the food nutritious? Is it prepared by a vendor who can offer quality and access guarantees or who can form a contract that reduces liability risk for the long-term care facility?	Is eating a communal experience that fosters connection and belonging? Do residents have real choices over what they eat? Could a resident share a cherished family recipe with kitchen staff?
Physical safety	Are the correct medications dispensed on time with the correct instructions? Are all fall risks minimized? Are residents with respiratory infections identified quickly enough to prevent communal transmission?	Are residents involved in designing their own physical safety care plan, and do they have the authority to define the appropriate balance between physical safety, possible risks, and autonomy? Do persons have enough privacy to build a space that they can identify with?
Social activities	Is there a full schedule of activities—bingo, mall visits—that ensures that residents are kept busy? Are these activities easy to monitor?	Do activities foster genuine connection and mutual understanding? Are there opportunities for residents to organize and lead social activities based on their own life skills and experiences? Do the activities serve some kind of social purpose—e.g., supporting charity—beyond simply keeping residents busy?
Health	Are appropriate standards of care being implemented and maintained for each resident, given their own medical history? Are any negative changes in health caught quickly enough?	Is the resident treated as a partner in decision-making about health? Are discussions about health framed so that the residents can easily express how their personal values interface with the facility's focus on health? Are emotional and spiritual well-being treated as components of good health? Is autonomy treated the same?

addressed in both the safety *and* the autonomy column will be a better place to live simply because such an institution will function as a much more effective stage in which its residents can express the principles of their lives—express, that is to say, their own autonomy.

Discussion and Reflection Questions

1. The chapter emphasizes the distinction between independence and autonomy. How does understanding this important difference impact how you would approach care planning for an older adult who expresses a desire to perform tasks independently, even if it is difficult or painful for them?
2. We have argued that "safety is not a first principle" for most people. How does this idea challenge common assumptions about what constitutes "good care" for older adults, and what are the implications for balancing safety concerns with a person's values and identity?
3. We have contrasted "desires" with "principles" when considering a person's values. How can healthcare professionals move beyond simply addressing a person's immediate desires to uncover and support their deeper life principles, and what might this look like in a practical care setting?

Reference

Majercsik E (2005) Hierarchy of needs of geriatric patients. Gerontology 51(3):170–173. https://doi.org/10.1159/000083989

How Prioritizing Safety Can Backfire

6

6.1 Case Illustration

Ed and Grace Leavitt have been married for 61 years. Dr. Grace Leavitt (age 84) was a retired professor of Renaissance Literature from the University of Michigan. She enjoyed a long and successful academic career, was widely published, and was a much sought-after lecturer in her professional circles. Mr. Ed Leavitt was a stay-at-home dad and relished his role, especially since it was such a novel situation for a man at that time. Prior to marrying Grace, Ed worked for one of the major auto manufacturers on the assembly line and hated the tedium of that position. Staying home to tend to the children and hone his cooking skills was a welcome relief for Ed and allowed Grace to engage fully in her academic career. Ed and Grace have two adult children, a daughter, Andrea, an architect who lives in Colorado with her wife, Danisha, and a son, Simon, who is a physician and married to Maria and lives in Minnesota with their two children.

Ed and Grace have enjoyed a life of travel, culture, and community engagement. They have lived in a community known for alternative points of view and have been active in politics. Their home has been full of books, music, and friends and has always been cluttered. Ed and Grace have always been night owls. It had been their habit to watch the late shows and then, at around two in the morning, go shopping at the local supermarket because it was so quiet in the middle of the night.

*On a recent visit to see his parents, Simon was appalled at the condition of their home and their health. The home, a large four-bedroom, two-story house in Ann Arbor was a shambles and in need of long overdue maintenance (*e.g.*, painting, overgrown trees and shrubs,* etc.*). Stacks of books and papers were piled onto every available surface. The cat's litter box had not been emptied in over a week. Ed, who has advanced Parkinson's disease, had a laceration over his left eye from a recent fall and was unkempt, needing a shave and haircut, his sweater soiled with food from lunch. Simon was shocked to see that his mother's dementia was much more advanced than he had discerned through their periodic phone conversations. She*

T. A. Harvath, M. Fedyk, *What If Maslow Was Wrong?*,
https://doi.org/10.1007/978-3-032-14249-8_6

takes medication for her type II diabetes but couldn't remember how often she was to take it. Simon was particularly concerned when he realized that his mother was still driving. Ed tried to reassure his son that he was always with Grace when they went out and served as her "navigator and copilot."

Simon immediately enlisted the help of his sister to pressure their parents to move closer to Simon so that he could monitor their status more closely. Ed and Grace were reluctant to give up their home but were persuaded that they would have more opportunities to see their two grandchildren if they were closer. Although Ed and Grace were willing to leave most of their furniture behind, they could not part with their books and the art and memorabilia they had collected during their years of international travel. Consequently, they arrived in their one-bedroom assisted living apartment with stacks of boxes that filled the living space and bedroom, making it difficult to maneuver easily around the small apartment.

Ed and Grace's story is familiar to anyone who has tried to help aging parents from afar. It's not unusual for adult children to only get part of the story when talking on the phone. It isn't until they visit that they see the decline in both the living conditions and the health of their parents. When these situations arise, we often see only two alternatives: #1 try to support them in their current living situation by visiting more often and rallying whatever local supports might be available, or #2 uproot them from their communities, and move them closer so that they can be monitored more closely. As we consider these two options under the self-imposed pressure of coming to a decision quickly, we tend to view moving them closer as the better, safer, more convenient option, without full comprehension of the risks that such a move can entail.

This choice is a perfect illustration of the nature of an impossible choice. Both options under consideration have serious downsides and important upsides, but there is not a logical rule or body of scientific studies that would tell Ed and Grace exactly how to weigh those risks and benefits. There are hundreds of books (including this one!) that Grace and Ed's children could read: but none of this erases the fact that a choice needs to be made (even if the choice is to stay put), and the consequences of that choice will have to be faced by not just Ed and Grace and their children but also by whoever else ends up getting involved in the situation. Impossible choices require courage, careful discernment, and often more time than we allow.

We've observed that many families, when faced with an impossible choice like this, feel that choice #2 is better than choice #1 because #2 feels like more of a choice: selecting it means doing *something* rather than accepting the persistence of a status quo that seems emotionally untenable. Choice #2 may also seem to make the situation more controllable and therefore make it easier for Andrea and Simon to spring into action to address any unforeseen emergency. It is easy to understand why choice #2 seemed like the right choice for the Leavitt's.

As the weeks went by, Ed and Grace continued to rifle through the boxes in their apartment, but they never seemed to make much headway. Papers were everywhere. Open boxes still contained unwrapped contents. Simon started getting phone calls from Marcella Winthrop, the administrator at the assisted living facility. Ms. Winthrop was concerned that the boxes in Ed and Grace's apartment posed both a fire risk and a risk for falls. She wanted Simon to urge his parents to get the boxes unpacked and removed from the apartment. Simon was frustrated because he and his wife had both tried to get his parents to downsize before they moved to no avail. Now that they were moved into assisted living, he had hoped that the staff there would help with that project and save him from further confrontation.

Another reason that making choices like #2 can seem attractive is that these choices help manage the "risk budget" inherent in any complex social situation. In Ed and Grace's case, Simon believed that he might be able to offload some of the risk management tasks to the facility. In contrast, Marcella had a keen sense of the impact that Ed and Grace's move was having on her facility's ability to manage its risks. Marcella's job involves allocating scarce resources to all sorts of different goals and needs. Rarely are there resources sufficient to satisfy *all* these goals and needs, so Marcella must figure out what should be prioritized, and usually the most rational thing for a manager in her position to do is to try to address the largest risks to the operational stability of the facility but if only doing so were as easy as just adding up and ranking the risks and then dedicating time or money and responsibility to addressing the most severe of the risks. In Marcella's mind, it is the family who should shoulder some of the responsibility for risk management.

At this point, the research of the psychologist Paul Slovic is helpful. He has spent several decades studying the ways in which we perceive risks and has paid particular attention to how perceptions of risk can come apart from objective risk. Simplifying some of his studies (Slovic et al. 2016; Slovic 2016), he argues that two attributes of risks can sometimes make them appear larger than they really are—the *dread factor* and the *uncertainty factor*. The dread factor refers to the tendency to believe that something is very risky if it seems to us to have catastrophic potential, no matter how low the objective probability of catastrophe is. The uncertainty factor refers to the tendency to believe that something is very risky if it seems like it is out of our control or ability to actively monitor—again, no matter how low the objective probability of catastrophe is. A risk that has the characteristics of both the dread factor and the uncertainty factor is a risk that is unlikely to be reasoned through objectivity.

Unfortunately, from Marcella's perspective, the pile of boxes cluttering Ed and Grace's apartment has those two factors: there is a chance (of unknown probability) that a serious injury could occur because of slipping on some papers or being knocked over by an off-balance box that then falls. From the perspective of Simon and Andrea, the pile of boxes carries a lot of uncertainty: even though the boxes are now closer, being stacked up in Minnesota rather than in Michigan where they were spread throughout the house, they are just as hard to monitor now as they were from afar. Ed and Grace's children may agree with Marcella that the "risk budget" that is associated with Ed and Grace's situation has increased, perhaps substantially so. But they don't agree on whose responsibility it is to manage this increased risk. They may think that another choice like #2 needs to be made, in order to manage these new risks. Doing "something" can seem like a risk management strategy, but often it is just the illusion of risk management.

But, here, we get to an important point. From the perspective of Ed and Grace, nothing significant has changed in terms of the risks both are facing as they go about their lives. The house in Michigan was just as cluttered. It also had additional hazards like unmanaged cat litter. If Grace or Ed were to suffer a serious fall, it would probably be harder for them to get help in Michigan rather than in Minnesota (at least harder for Simon and Andrea to respond to and stay on top of the situation). The big change, here, is that the objective risks that Ed and Grace face are now more *salient* to the people who are trying to care for them: Marcella, Andrea, and Simon. Because Ed and Grace's living situation is now within the control or, at least influence, of these three people, they are more aware of their limited ability to manage the "risk budget" that Ed and Grace's habits, choices, values, and preferences create.

But this observation shows that everyone involved in the care of Ed and Grace is still in the grip of an impossible choice. Electing to go with #2 did not really change the fundamental fact that there is no way around the risks—many of which are quite serious—that Ed and Grace face.

Several months have gone by, and Ed and Grace seemed to be settling into their new space, re-establishing the routines that they'd had in Michigan. Enough of the boxes have been unpacked so that they don't represent an ongoing concern for Marcella or Simon. Ed and Grace started doing the laundry together—they would load up the laundry basket and put it on Ed's lap as he sat on the wheelchair, and Grace would push him down the hall to the laundry room, where he would instruct her to load the washer, put in the detergent, and get the load going. Sometimes, they would forget about the laundry, much to the consternation of their new neighbors in assisted living, and leave the machines tied up for several hours.

Ed had insisted that they bring their car to Minnesota so that they could have some measure of independence and not be "cooped up" in the facility or dependent on Simon for transportation. Simon had decided not to push that issue and assumed that after they moved his mother would not be able to pass the test to get a Minnesota license and then they could sell the car. Unfortunately, Ed and Grace did not see any urgency in getting licensed in Minnesota and kept telling Simon that they would get to it as soon as things settled down.

Ed and Grace also continued to go grocery shopping in the middle of the night—something the staff complained about regularly. Sometimes, they would get lost getting to and from the store and would be gone for several hours. The staff worried that something may have happened to them and they would get blamed for any harm that came to the aged couple. When Ed and Grace did return to the facility, they often made a lot of noise as they loaded their bags onto the elevator and carried them down the hall. Other residents complained of the noise and asked that there be rules about quiet hours.

Again, Marcella called on Simon to reason with his parents and tell them they needed to shop during the day or go with the facility van that took other residents shopping on a weekly basis. Ed and Grace flatly refused to give up their nighttime escapades. They had no desire to go in a van with "all those old people." Simon felt caught in the middle. He pleaded with his sister to step in and help with this, but Andrea didn't see why her parents couldn't keep their car and refused to get involved.

These sorts of disagreements are common by-products of a situation defined by the persistent presence of an impossible choice. These disagreements do not have easy, obvious, or singular solutions that can satisfy all parties involved: there is no way to reason around or through them. Instead, they become a source of stress, seemingly endless family negotiations and conflicts, and eventually breakdowns in trust and cooperation.

But the story, at this point, also reveals something new. One of the ways that a risk budget gets managed is the creation of rules—both justified and arbitrary—the aim of which is to change the behavior of older adults so that the risk budget becomes more balanced. In effect, some of the older adult's autonomy is exchanged ("spent"!) for a marginal increase in perceived (not necessarily actual) safety.

Of course, there were rules back in Michigan for Ed and Grace—like "Do the grocery shopping at 2 am." Those rules are formed by long-standing patterns in Grace and Ed's life: for reasons that we discussed in the previous chapter, they express some of the married couple's deepest values. "Do the grocery shopping at 2 am" really is a principle of their lives. It was how they expressed their autonomy by creating rituals that gave them pleasure and meaning.

Unfortunately, it was not seen that way by Marcella and the assisted living staff. Ed and Grace were failing to adapt to the reality of their new social situation, and so new rules were being invented that had nothing to do with Ed and Grace's values to create a situation with a bit more control or order. These rules are not congruent with the principles of Ed and Grace's life, so not only are they living in a situation in which they may not be objectively safer than they were in their home in Michigan; they are starting to have their autonomy undermined by the creation of rules with little value congruence for Ed and Grace.

We want to suggest, therefore, that it would be an interesting exercise to ask if Marcella and her staff also tried to manage a "quality-of-life" budget alongside the "risk budget" that we have been talking about so far. The fact that Marcella's staff were worried about losing their jobs *because* Ed and Grace were acting autonomously suggests that the institution placed too much priority on safety. Imagine what a difference could be made if staff felt that they would be rewarded by contributing to the "quality-of-life" budget rather than punished: this would give some staff reason, perhaps, to find ways to help Ed and Grace with their laundry or their nightly grocery shopping.

Simon's wife Marie stepped in and offered to take Ed and Grace grocery shopping as part of a luncheon outing with the grandchildren. That solution delighted Ed and Grace and curtailed some, although not all, of their middle-of-the-night endeavors. However, just when it seemed that things had finally settled down, Simon got a call from Ms. Winthrop regarding Ed's "unsafe" ambulation. Ed's Parkinson's disease created challenges for his mobility at times. Sometimes, he needed a wheelchair to get around; other times, a cane or walker would help steady his gait. However, Ed did not like to use the cane or walker and tended to "surf" the furniture in their apartment to get around. He would walk, laying a hand on tables, chairs, or bookcases (and boxes), to move about the apartment. And while this worked in their tiny, crowded apartment, it did not work well in the hallways and common areas of the facility. Still, Ed resisted using the walker. The staff tried to tell Ed he could not walk in the hallways unless he had his walker or standby assistance, but Ed continued to walk around without assistance. He had fallen a couple of times, skinning his knee, bruising his elbow, but had not sustained a serious injury, so he tended to be dismissive of staff concerns.

One day, Ed lost his balance in the community room and fell into another resident, causing her to fall and break her hip. Ms. Winthrop called an urgent family conference and informed Simon, Ed, and Grace that the facility was implementing specific guidelines for Ed and Grace that they would be required to adhere to or would face eviction. These guidelines included the following:

- *A 10 pm curfew. They would need to be back in the facility by 10 pm, or they would not be allowed in.*
- *Restrictions in movement in the common areas. Ed was only allowed to be in the common areas if he was in a wheelchair or using his walker.*
- *Laundry room schedule. Ed and Grace were assigned days/times for their laundry. They would not be allowed to use the machines outside of those times.*

Simon was furious. He was angry with his parents for causing such upheaval in their facility and angry with the facility for not doing a better job of managing his parent's eccentricities. He was also worried that his parents would face eviction or a lawsuit for causing the other woman's injury or both. He began to wonder whether he had made a mistake in forcing his parents to move. Afterall, they were not really safer in this facility, and their care became much more complex, even though they were closer geographically.

Simon's question is of course the main point of this story: it turns out that Ed and Grace probably weren't any safer in the facility than at home. Picking choice #2 had not really changed any of the fundamental properties of Grace and Ed's situation. They were both losing their capabilities, but their values and their connection were still intact. Moving Ed and Grace into the assisted living facility in Minnesota had not slowed the aging process, and it certainly did not change the Leavitt's stubborn willingness to continue to live their lives according to their values. In reality, it added additional stress and complexity to a situation that was already stressful and complex—the impossibility of the situation was unchanged.

6.2 Case Discussion

There are three big points that we want to make in our discussion of this case. The first is that there is a temptation to see this story as a series of errors that simply compounded until someone really did get hurt, and the Leavitt family was starting to lose its integrity. However, this is not the most constructive way to look at this case, and not just because it invites the temptation to pass judgment or assign blame. The reason is more subtle: if there really has been an error, then there must have, at the time a particular decision was made, been some reason to make a different decision, and the error, therefore, was partly a lack of awareness or sensitivity to those reasons. This is why, when we apologize for an error, we find ourselves saying "Sorry—I should have paid more attention to that!" When a family is in the grip of an impossible choice, however, there really is no "right" or no "wrong" choice: there are just choices that must be selected, which will bring consequences and risks no matter what. Families cannot make erroneous choices when they are in the grip of an impossible choice. We truly cannot say that it would have been better for Ed and Grace to remain in Michigan because we cannot know what challenges would have arisen for them there: those sorts of conclusions aren't justified, no matter how much hindsight we get, when a family faces an impossible choice.

The second point is the importance of one of Terri's favorite questions, a question to ask prior to placement: "What are you hoping will happen with this move?" Or: "For what problem is the move a solution?" Sometimes, when families make the choice to move older parents into assisted living facilities, they almost always assume that the older adult will be safer than in their current situation. They may also assume that the change in location is going to lead to deep changes in character or that there will be greater control over the situation. But older adults are people too: they will always find a way of expressing themselves no matter the situation. There is consequently some wisdom in thinking about how to find a living arrangement that does not put a couple like Ed and Grace in a position where they must go to unreasonable extremes to express themselves. But there are two deeper issues that Terri's questions raise that we want to make:

- First, no matter how hard we try, we cannot protect older adults from all the bad things that could happen to them. It does not mean that we should be cavalier about concerns for their safety and disregard risks. Instead, we need to delve into the risks, try to understand their likelihood of happening, and explore what can be done to mitigate those risks and try to clarify the impact of those efforts on the older adult's quality of life and autonomy. And we can't assume that the alternatives are risk-free. It is impossible to expect that nursing homes or assisted living facilities can offer risk-free living and if they could it would likely be the sort of life that isn't really living.
- Second, it is unreasonable to expect dramatic changes from people, young or old: for most of us, our personality, our values, our habits, and our connections are rather enduring, even stubbornly unchanging! This is not necessarily the best thing, morally speaking. The world would be a better place if we could more effortlessly overcome our shortcomings and imperfections. Yet, we are as we are, and situations of impossible choice cannot be dissolved by hoping that someone's parents or partners will become more flexible and adaptable, more reasonable, and more safety-focused, when their health and functional status change. The one thing that you can count on when dealing with an impossible choice is that everyone involved—parents, siblings, friends, cousins, nursing facility staff—is probably going to remain the person that they were before the impossible choice showed its ugly face. Stubborn people don't become more adapt-

able, social butterflies don't become silent introverts, and risk-takers don't suddenly become more cautious.

The third and final point in this section gets us back to how to think about safety. When families are faced with choices like that between #1 and #2, they rely on an idealized view of what safety means. Safety is what can be controlled systematically: a "risk budget" can be formed so that the most immediate and most serious risks are always identified and managed. But as our comments about rules above, suggestion, along with the "risk budgets," comes a system of vigilance and control that slowly degrades autonomy. But it is not only autonomy that is degraded; happiness also suffered in this story. Ed and Grace's experiences starkly illustrate one of the biggest paradoxes in ethics: that a singular focus on safety can be inadvertently self-undermining. By opting for choice #2, the Leavitt family ultimately found themselves in a situation where rules were imposed upon Ed and Grace that negatively impacted their well-being and the stress and disagreements among the family and the assisted living staff negatively impacted the well-being of the entire family. Aggregate happiness probably decreased in this story, as a direct result of perusing safety.

The story of Ed and Grace should help us think very carefully about the foundations of care of older adults. Pursuing a "safety first" or even a "safety above all else" agenda may precipitate a series of conflicts and even crises that harm the autonomy and the quality of life of everyone involved in any case. In short, cases like this should make us think that, yes, probably, the interpretation of Maslow we discussed back in Chap. 1 was wrong—safety should not be the only thing we focus on when making decisions about old age care. Balancing concerns of safety with autonomy and quality of life is simple and less taxing way of dealing with an impossible choice. Remember, though, the goal shouldn't be to design a three-legged safety, autonomy, and quality-of-life stool with absolutely no wobble whatsoever. Instead, the goal should instead make sure the stool doesn't completely tip over.

Discussion and Reflection Questions

1. Like in past chapters, this chapter argues for the perspective that "impossible choices" in care of older adults have no objectively "right" or "wrong" answers. How might understanding this perspective influence how you approach difficult decisions with patients and their families, especially when safety is a primary concern?
2. The "dread factor" and "uncertainty factor" are introduced as ways our perception of risk can differ from objective risk. Can you recall a situation (either personal or professional) where these factors might have influenced your or someone else's assessment of a situation's risk? How could you try to account for these biases in your future practice?
3. The concept of a "quality-of-life" budget is proposed alongside a "risk budget." In what ways could healthcare settings actively manage and prioritize a "quality-

of-life" budget for older adults, and what challenges might arise in implementing such an approach?

4. We have suggested that individuals, including older adults, are often stubbornly unchanging in their personality, values, and habits. How does this idea challenge the expectation that moving an older adult to a new care environment will fundamentally alter their behaviors or preferences? What implications does this have for person-centered care?

References

Slovic P (2016) The perception of risk. Earthscan risk in society. Routledge

Slovic P, Fischhoff B, Lichtenstein S (2016) Facts and fears: understanding perceived risk. In: The Perception of Risk. Routledge

7 Sex and the Nursing Home

7.1 Case Illustration

Hannah and Fred Picard had been living independently in a continuing care retirement community for several years. Married for over 60 years, they each had significant health problems that were starting to erode their ability to maintain themselves and their apartment. Hannah, 91, had type II diabetes and peripheral vascular disease and had undergone bilateral below-the-knee amputations because of chronic, nonhealing wounds that extended to mid-calf. She had mild dementia and frequent bouts of delirium related to the infections, surgery, and fluctuating blood glucose levels. Fred, 93, had a long history of alcohol abuse but was devoted to Hannah and tried to care for her as best he could. Hannah was admitted to a skilled nursing facility following a recent revision of her right stump, and Fred visited every day, helping Hannah with meals and wheeling her around the facility to visit different residents they both knew.

In the afternoon, Hannah would take a nap, and Fred would return to their apartment for a few hours. When he returned to help Hannah for dinner, the staff could smell alcohol on his breath, and his gait was often unstable. One day, Fred didn't return for the evening meal and Hannah grew worried. The staff checked on Fred and found that he had fallen in his apartment and fractured his hip. Fred was taken to the hospital where he had surgical repair of the fracture, and he was admitted to the skilled nursing facility for rehabilitation. Initially, Fred and Hannah were in different rooms, waiting for a double room to open so they could be together. The staff ensured that they ate together at meals and had the opportunity to kiss goodnight before helping each of them to bed at night.

Soon after Fred's admission, it was clear that his mental status had undergone significant decline during his hospitalization. He had independent wheelchair mobility (using his legs to propel the wheelchair), and he soon started

T. A. Harvath, M. Fedyk, *What If Maslow Was Wrong?*,
https://doi.org/10.1007/978-3-032-14249-8_7

wandering into the rooms of other residents, causing much distress to those residents. When Fred was helped into bed, he often started masturbating, seemingly unaware that staff and his roommate were in the room. The staff responded by trying to give Fred privacy, timing his bedtime routine so that he was in bed before his roommate.

One night, Hannah was being wheeled into Fred's room to kiss him goodnight, and she saw him masturbating. She didn't quite understand what was happening, and she expressed great concern that he was having a seizure. The nursing assistant tried to reassure Hannah that he wasn't having a seizure but was reluctant to tell her what was happening, unsure of how to explain masturbation to a slightly confused 91-year-old woman. The RN on duty was asked to speak with Hannah. The nurse tried to explain to Hannah that Fred was masturbating, but Hannah didn't seem to understand. Hannah expressed concern that perhaps she wasn't fulfilling her spousal duties if Fred needed to masturbate. The nurse asked Hannah if she wanted to have some privacy with Fred so that they could have sex, and Hannah declined. She admitted that she never really enjoyed sex and would be embarrassed that the staff would know what she and Fred were doing behind closed doors.

When a double room opened up, Fred and Hannah were moved in together. It caused immediate challenges for the staff. Fred continued to masturbate when in bed, and Hannah continued to fear that Fred was having seizures or was in need of something, putting on the call light and summoning staff to a room where Fred was still masturbating. Repeated explanations and reassurances failed to soothe Hannah's concerns. They tried simply pulling the curtain between the two beds at night, but Fred's masturbation caused the bed to creak, and the noise was distressing to Hannah. The staff debated how to resolve this ongoing issue. Should they separate the couple even though Hannah was not in favor of that option (Fred was not able to express his wishes due to his cognitive impairment, replying "yes" when asked whether he wanted to stay with Hannah or be moved to another room).

7.2 Dealing with the Loss of Rational Capacity

Clearly, Fred's efforts to comfort or pleasure himself present difficulties for both Hannah and the staff of the nursing home. Since these difficulties are quite different, we will discuss them separately. So, let us start with the staff of the nursing home. There are two strategies that can help the staff make decisions when dealing with cases like Fred's. The first involves a principle which can easily be justified within a Kantian framework that builds on ideas we introduced previously. The second involves a different kind of principle—one that we will explain in some detail because this new principle can be a powerful source of cooperation between nursing home staff, residents like Hannah, and any family members who get involved in the care of residents or patients like Hannah and Friend.

7.3 Retained Humanity

The Kantian principle first, then. This is the idea that people like Fred who, despite their lack of decisional capacity, have nevertheless "retained humanity" (Kant 2020). His severe dementia means that he is no longer making rational choices for himself. Still, it does not mean that everyone else in Fred's life is free to treat him however they want. Instead, the principle of "retained humanity" refers to Fred's intrinsic worth as a person. And while he might lack the ability to rationally evaluate and then decide what principles motivate his actions, most of the people involved in Fred's life can work together to make ethical choices about Fred. These choices can be informed by Fred's needs for comfort, self-expression—and the fact that, despite his dementia (and even because of it), Fred is still a unique person with unique feelings and a life history of choice that form deep patterns. While Fred's nightly activities might not meet the ethical standards of a rational choice, his masturbation can still be respected as an expression of his remaining self or even as an expression of patterns of life (remember Chap. 5), and the nursing home staff can therefore explore different ways of helping Fred "retain his humanity." In fact, it seems that the nursing home staff is already motivated by something like this principle. Why? In concrete terms, a strategy that helps Fred retain his humanity would be a strategy very similar to what the nursing home staff attempted. Let's explore this in more details.

Privacy Fred's activities would probably only be ethical (at least according to the Kantian framework) if they were done in privacy, so the nursing home staff can help Fred "retain his humanity" by exploring how to make Fred's space more private—perhaps with a room divider or a bed canopy. By taking any of these steps, the nursing home staff still treat Fred as a person with a right to privacy, rather than an object whose behavior must be monitored or even controlled. And while Fred's behavior might not be rationally intentional, what he is doing is still deeply personal—and so any small steps that increase Fred's privacy also facilitate his self-soothing or physical release in ways that are aligned with choices that he might have made for himself in the past.

Deep Clinical Assessment It is not clear from the story above *why* Fred is touching himself whenever he goes to bed. This is an opportunity to leverage the clinical resources of the nursing home for Fred's benefit. A thorough physical assessment, observational routines, and deep dive into Fred's family history may reveal potential triggers or underlying needs that are directly connected to Fred's behavior. For example, it could reveal that Fred has synesthesia which leads to sensory overload when he is falling asleep, and Fred's masturbation has been an effective strategy for calming his senses down so that he can sleep. This of course is a hypothetical suggestion, but, even so, it means that calming music, darkening the lights before starting Fred's bedtime routine, or giving Fred a weighted blanket may reduce the need for Fred to touch himself. As before, these might be actions that Fred would choose for himself were he capable of understanding—and even being able to explain to nursing home staff—the role that masturbation plays in his life.

Advocate for New Policies Nursing home policies and resources ultimately exist for the benefit of residents. The rooming policy at the nursing home—who gets single rooms versus who gets double rooms—is of course ultimately under the control of the nursing home management. Fred will probably not be the only resident who presents complex needs and challenges; sexual needs and capacities do not disappear with the onset of dementia. Nursing home staff might therefore be able to argue that a policy covering sexually active patients with dementia include prioritizing giving these patients single rooms. As before, this might be a choice that Fred would make for himself, but here is an interesting twist. A policy that prioritizes giving sexually active patients with dementia single rooms might be a policy that almost everyone connected with the nursing home—residents, patients, families, staff, and administration—would choose because of how it supports everyone's autonomy. Everyone might be freer to be themselves if such a policy were adopted. So, not only would such a policy help Fred retain his humanity; it would also help everyone else at the nursing home express theirs.

7.4 Experiments in Living

Kantian principles are intellectually attractive. They align with common beliefs about agency and intentionality and very elegantly express the moral intuition that the basis of any moral or ethical action cannot be a rule that applies only to a single individual or only in a highly specific, perhaps totally-one-of-a-kind situation. But Kantian principles are nevertheless still very abstract, and that makes it hard to be certain that they are truly applied in real-world circumstances. Because of this, we want to analyze Fred's case using a different perspective that has its roots in the pragmatist tradition in ethics.

The core of ethical pragmatism is the following rule for making choices and taking actions: Without making things worse, try to discover how to make things better (Fedyk 2022). This "rule" can be put into practice by treating ethical problems as opportunities to experimentally implement practices that are routine in most clinical settings in order to discover the effects of different practices. Amongst clinicians, doing this is sometimes referred to as "quality improvement" or "patient safety". What we are suggesting here is that these practices can be extended to discover novel solutions to ethical dilemmas like what to do about Fred's nightly activities.

Here is the idea in more detail. Putting the pragmatic principle *without making things worse, try to discover how to make things better* normally will entail the following:

- Focus on small, incremental changes that have easy-to-observe effects. Avoid any drastic overhauls or systematic changes if possible. Avoid the assumption that whatever change is made it cannot be reversed if it makes things worse.
- Observe as much as possible. Carefully monitor both the effects of changes and what sorts of things are unaffected by any of the small changes.

- Plan subsequent changes based upon careful analysis of the first round of small, incremental changes. Be open to reverse any changes that appear to make things worse, and try to discover how to incrementally strengthen or stabilize any positive (even if quite small) effects with any subsequent changes. All changes, though, should continue to be small and incremental.
- Don't worry about definitions of big concepts like "good," "morally correct," and so on. These concepts cannot easily describe the effects of small changes: instead, try to carefully observe ways the changes do in fact cause improvements ("make things better") or do not cause improvements (either have no effect or "make things worse"). Evidence of relative small changes internal to the situation will usually be more than enough information to make critical ethical choices about that situation.
- Be creative, adaptable, and flexible—prioritize learning about a situation rather than getting things right with every choice or change. It is hard to know in advance what sorts of change will or won't be effective at making things better without making things worse. It is therefore OK to make a small change with the expectation that they may lead to an improvement, discover that in fact the change makes things worse, then reverse the change, and come away from the situation with an improved understanding of its causal structure. This will drive deeper learning about the situation, increasing the ability to identify future changes that do in fact make things better without making anything worse.
- The clinical goal is an easy-to-describe, easy-to-communicate "model" of a situation that describes what sorts of things either cause or stabilize "better effects" and what sorts of things help avoid "worse effects."

These strategies are routinely used by physicians and nurses to figure out how to care for patients. What is novel here is the suggestion that these strategies can be extended to support ethical decision-making. So, let us illustrate these ideas by returning to Fred and Hannah's situation. We'll intentionally use strategies that mirror the concrete suggestions above, so that the differences emerge in the detail.

Incremental Privacy Fred's tendency to touch himself emerges most prominently shortly after he goes to bed. A pragmatic strategy might be to incrementally add more privacy to Fred's situation—starting with room dividers, putting him to bed earlier than Hannah, extending to more complex options like giving him a moveable bed, and allowing him to fall asleep in a nearby observation room before wheeling him into his overnight room—and observe the effects of any of these changes for 2 or 3 days. Perhaps a different bed that didn't creak as much could help. It may be possible to discover just the right combination of privacy-supporting resources and practices that resolve most of the friction caused by the situation. Alternatively, nursing home staff may discover that there is no practical way of giving Fred enough privacy to avoid upsetting Hannah or disturbing Fred's roommates.

Incremental Alternatives to Self-Pleasuring This proposal assumes that Fred is motivated at some level to comfort or sooth himself as he is falling asleep. With the help of Hannah, nursing home staff could try placing objects that are familiar to Fred in his bed before he goes to sleep, exploring whether, for instance, a particular blanket or pillow is attractive to Fred as a source of comfort or soothing. Alternatively, nursing home staff could develop a multi-week plan of "micro-adjustments' to Fred nighttime routine—such as dimming the lights earlier than normal, giving Fred a back rub before putting him to bed (perhaps with the assistance of Hannah), playing some of Fred's favorite music, or telling him a story until he falls asleep. It might be possible to swaddle Fred in bed to give him a sense of comfort that would be soothing. As before, the suggestion would be to try any of these potential comfort objects or micro-adjustments for several days, carefully observing whether they make any difference to Fred's behavior. There is a small chance that they moderate or even completely suppress Fred's urge to touch himself; there is an even greater chance that they provide Fred some comfort independent of his nightly activities. Either way, this approach is likely to generate useful information about Fred, because if none of the soothing objects makes a difference to either Fred's urges or his more general emotional welfare, then this itself is a useful information that can be used to learn how to care better for Fred, both connected to his masturbation specifically and also other elements of his care.

Staff Attitudes and Responses The pragmatic approach does not require that we focus only on interventions that directly impact patients or residence. Absolutely any element of a care situation can be the focus of experimental, incremental changes—after all, the reason to try to discover how to make things better without making things worse is that we simply don't know what sorts of actions or choices do or do not make a positive difference in the situation. Thus, in Fred's case, how the staff react to Fred's behaviors can itself be a source of learning. A nurse manager might organize a brief, target huddle with a small number of night staff team members in which Fred's masturbation behaviors are described not as "problems" that need to be stopped or suppressed but rather as Fred communicating his needs and emotional states. Staff can use this orientation to learn more about the immediate conditions surrounding Fred's behavior, looking to observe and learn before potentially intervening and reacting.

Framing Fred's behavior as an effort to communicate and the staff acting as detectives to try to learn what Fred is saying help everyone avoid making decisions about Fred based on mistaken assumptions. Staff can be asked to record exactly *when* Fred starts and stops his activities (e.g., immediately after going to bed, sometimes as long as 20 minutes after lights out, only on days where he was wakeful the night before, or every single day), *how* Fred seems while he is touching himself (e.g., agitated, distracted, unaware, relaxed, focused, sleepy, alert), and what seems to precede it (e.g., a heavy meal, seeing Hannah, being confused about something in his past, the appearance of loneliness). It is possible that these observations eventually coalesce together into a story that explains why it is that Fred is touching himself, a story that might provide insight about how to change the situation for everyone's benefit, for instance, perhaps Fred self-pleasures less on days when he sees Hannah only in the afternoon and not immediately before bed, or maybe working with his favorite aide tends to increase the frequency of his activities.

7.5 Consent

We trust that you have noticed some of the overlap between the Kantian and the pragmatist approach to learning how to treat Fred ethically. That is normal: it is usually the case that different ethical frameworks offer similar advice and guidance when they are thoughtfully applied to any case.

There is, however, an important set of problems where the Kantian framework should always be the default and only abandoned in favor of an alternative framework with exceptionally strong reason. The set is composed of any problems that involve sexual connection between people, where the goal is to ensure that any such connection is always consensual. What this means, ethically, is that everyone involved in the sexual activity should be aware of their reasons for participating in the activity and accept those reasons as sufficient to justify their choice to continue participating in the action. In other words, sexual activities should always be consensual, which means they must always be intentional, in the ethical sense above.

Practically, then, this means that nursing home staff should be very cautious about facilitating or allowing sexual contact between partners with dementia. Sufficiently advanced dementia removes the ability of one or both partners to consent to the activity. As we've explored with Fred's masturbation, this means that connections between people with dementia may not actually be, technically, sexual acts if they cannot consent to them. But at a deeper level, the actions may fall into an ambiguous gray zone in between intentional and non-intentional actions, in which it is not possible to determine whether consent does or does not exist. It is probably better to explore alternatives—including masturbation or something like that—when presented with a grey zone scenario.

7.6 Back to Safety

Finally, we want to bring our discussion back to one of the main themes of this book, safety. What we've tried to show in this analysis of Fred's situation is how two different ethical frameworks—the Kantian ideal as expressed in "retained humanity" and the pragmatist approach consisting of "trying to discover how to make things better without making things worse"—can be used to think through morally complex cases. Neither places any central or essential importance on safety, even though both allow considerations of safety to play an important, potentially even decisive role. What this means, then, is that the two ethical frameworks that we have explored in this chapter help answer the question "What are some alternatives to the ethical framework 'maximize safety' that can be used to make decisions about care?" The Kantian framework and the pragmatist frameworks are attractive alternatives, and if you are especially interested in exploring a case in your own life, what Fred and Hannah's story shows is that both can be applied in a complementary fashion.

Discussion and Reflection Questions

1. The concept of "retained humanity" suggests that even individuals with severe dementia still have intrinsic worth as people. How can healthcare professionals ensure they are treating patients with dementia as individuals with retained humanity, even when their behaviors are challenging or difficult to understand?
2. The chapter introduces the idea of "experiments in living" as a way to address ethical dilemmas, focusing on small, observable changes that incrementally improve a patient's situation. Imagine a challenging situation with an older adult patient where you are unsure of the best course of action. How could you apply the method of "without making things worse, try to discover how to make things better" to find a solution?
3. Why is consent particularly complex and important when considering sexual activity for older adults with advanced dementia? What are some practical ways that nursing home staff can navigate these sensitive situations in a way that preserves everyone's integrity (including the integrity of the staff)?

References

Fedyk M (2022) How philosophy of science can unlock new methods in bioethics. Am J Bioeth: AJOB 22:51. Taylor & Francis

Kant I (2020) Groundwork of the metaphysic of morals. In: Immanuel Kant: groundwork of the metaphysic of morals in focus. Routledge, pp 17–98

8 When Safety Matters Most to a Provider but Not the Older Adult

8.1 Case Illustration

Frank Waters, age 85, was admitted to the nursing home for rehabilitation after falling at home. He had been lying on the floor for a day and a half when his neighbor found him. Shortly after admission, the interdisciplinary team recognized that severe dementia was preventing him from reaping the full benefits of physical and occupational therapy. He stood without locking his wheelchair; he wandered away from his walker; he tried to get out of bed without assistance. Consequently, he fell, repeatedly. The team held a family conference to discuss discharge plans. Ahead of the family conference, the social worker confirmed with Mr. Waters' sister that placement in a congregate care environment was a foregone conclusion. He was no longer safe living alone in his home.

During the family conference that included the entire interdisciplinary team, Mr. Waters, his sister, and two next-door neighbors, Mr. Waters sat silently with his head bowed and eyes closed while each team member took a turn presenting their assessments that would justify the recommendation for placement. After each team member had given their report, Mr. Waters was asked whether he wanted to say anything. He lifted his head, looked around the room, and said, loudly and clearly, "Three days on the floor in my home is worth more than 3 years in any nursing home you have!" He bowed his head again as everyone sat in stunned silence. Finally, his sister asked whether it was possible to send him home. His neighbors said that they could check on him once or twice a day. The social worker suggested a home healthcare aide to help with meals and bathing. Slowly, the team put together a plan for Mr. Waters to return to his home that included an emergency call button and some minor home modifications.

Then, the physical therapist voiced the collective concern that had been lurking just beneath the surface: "What are we thinking? Are we really going to send this man home? What kind of liability will we have when he falls and gets hurt? He is no longer safe at home!" In the end, we honored his request and sent him home with as

T. A. Harvath, M. Fedyk, *What If Maslow Was Wrong?*,
https://doi.org/10.1007/978-3-032-14249-8_8

much support as possible. We documented our decision, concluding that although we weren't ignoring his risk for injury from falling, we saw that the threat to the quality of his life was of greater concern in this situation.

8.2 Chapter Outline

When the needs for safety, quality of life, and autonomy clash, older adults often choose quality of life and autonomy over safety. Mr. Waters stated his choice succinctly, despite cognitive impairment, providing compelling direction for the staff. We cannot, however, always assume that older adults with dementia will be able to use a fleeting period of lucidity or focus to precisely articulate their values and preferences. All the same, as we have argued in previous chapters, it does not follow that these older persons do not have values and preferences. Clinical research is consistent with this position: Sharp and Bryant found that older persons with dysphagia sometimes choose textured foods, despite the risk of aspiration, because food plays such a central role in their lives (Sharp and Bryant 2003). Similarly, Yardley, Donovan-Hall, and Todd found that older adults at risk for falling resist home modifications (such as removing throw rugs) because they fear that such precautions will breed dependence (Yardley et al. 2006). While the onset of dementia or diminished physical capacities can change a person's risk profile, this research shows there still tends to be an overriding preference to maximize autonomy or quality of life over concerns for safety.

We should not assume, therefore, that as a person's ability to express or articulate their values diminishes, they start to value safety proportionally. It is also a mistake to reason that, because a person's capacities are diminishing, steps should be taken to preserve only the lowermost elements of Maslow's hierarchy. Even though the upper layers of the pyramid depend upon the lower layers, directing support toward only safety and basic needs does not automatically cause still living elements of the upper levels to shrivel—again, remember Mr. Kane's boysenberry pie!

But what should an older adult or a concerned family caregiver do when they are working with a provider—a physician, a social worker, a home health nurse, or really anyone who has some degree of power to determine how an older adult is cared for—and the provider believes that safety is the only consideration that really matters? It is extremely common for providers to make the assessment that older adults like Frank are "no longer safe at home"; how should we think about these cases? An implication of Chap. 4 is that families are very likely to encounter providers who feel they have no other choice than to put safety first.

This case is particularly pointed. Not only did Frank express his values, but he also expressed them in a way that made them easy to plug into the cost-benefit reasoning that very often drives decisions of liability. The physical therapist's concerns are entirely appropriate. However, as we described, with appropriate documentation of Frank's preferences, honoring his wishes is a course of action that poses no unusual liability concerns. Not all cases are as clear as Frank's or Mr. Kane's.

8.3 The Older Adult Safety Paradigm

So, let us start by trying to understand some of the most common reasons why providers care about safety. For many doctors and nurses, it was the publication in 1999 of an Institute of Medicine report called *To Err Is Human* (Institute of Medicine (US) Committee on Quality of Health Care in America 2000). We discussed this publication previously. It is an extremely detailed report—effectively a book—that launched what can accurately be called the contemporary "older patient safety paradigm" (Bates and Singh 2018). According to the authors of *To Err Is Human*, safety is defined as *freedom from accidental injury*. But even more interesting, the authors offer a definition of quality of care that breaks it down into only three components: care that is consistent with prevailing medical standards, customization, and safety. The authors argue that providers have a responsibility to balance all three of these when, for instance, developing care plans for people like Mr. Waters. However, the focus of the report is primarily to detail how systematic approaches to standardizing older person care, measuring and reporting medical errors, and, crucially, implementing safety protocols can help avoid preventable deaths.

As we noted previously, preventable deaths, and associated metrics for quality care, have since become some of the important institutional targets for organized healthcare systems. It is worth quoting the IOM report in some detail to understand the logic of prevention that they rely upon:

> Not all errors result in harm. Errors that do result in injury are sometimes called preventable adverse events. An adverse event is an injury resulting from a medical intervention, or in other words, it is not due to the underlying condition of the patient. While all adverse events result from medical management, not all are preventable (i.e., not all are attributable to errors). For example, if a patient has surgery and dies from an infection he or she got post-operatively, it is an adverse event. If analysis of the case reveals that the patient got the infection because of poor hand washing or instrument cleaning techniques by staff, the adverse event was preventable (attributable to an error of execution). But the analysis may conclude that no error occurred, and the patient would be presumed to have had a difficult surgery and recovery (not a preventable adverse event).
>
> Much can be learned from the analysis of errors. All adverse events resulting in serious injury or death should be evaluated to assess whether improvements in the delivery system can be made to reduce the likelihood of similar events occurring in the future. Errors that do not result in harm also represent an important opportunity to identify system improvements having the potential to prevent adverse events. Preventing errors means designing the health care system at all levels to make it safer. Building safety into processes of care is a more effective way to reduce errors than blaming individuals […] The focus must shift from blaming individuals for past errors to a focus on preventing future errors by designing safety into the system. This does not mean that individuals can be careless. People must still be vigilant and held responsible for their actions. But when an error occurs, blaming an individual does little to make the system safer and prevent someone else from committing the same error. (Institute of Medicine (US) Committee on Quality of Health Care in America 2000, 4–5)

Let us now pull this reasoning apart.

First, notice the phrase "delivery system." This assumes that protocols and processes by which care is delivery can be standardized—or at least sufficiently standardized so that they can be managed and analyzed for the difference they make in patient outcomes—and that every individual expected to implement those protocols and processes will do so in a standardized manner. If handwashing was not mandatory before surgery and so handwashing occurred only semi-randomly or not according to standardized processes, it would not be possible to analyze whether handwashing contributed to occurrences of postop infections.

Second, the authors explicitly shift the locus of moral responsibility from individual provider—nurses, doctors, social workers, pharmacists, nursing assistants—and their individual judgments to the delivery system itself. Safety is to be achieved by addressing the "processes of care" rather than by asking individual providers to regard safety as an important moral principle. As a result, good outcomes are seen as a by-product of designing good care systems and adherent staff. At the minimum, this would ensure a care delivery system that rarely if ever contributes to causing some well-known form of error. Unfortunately, we need only look at one of the most common "preventable errors" targeted by patient safety activities—falls—to realize that standardized processes cannot always deliver on the desired outcomes they seek to ensure.

Third, and finally, notice that something is an error if it is preventable. But the authors are working with two different concepts of preventable. Strictly speaking, almost anything bad that happens to a patient—whether it is someone like Mr. Waters or a female patient who is in their 30 s and hospitalized for abdominal pain likely connected to an abscessing appendix—is preventable because, strictly speaking, the world could have been very different at some past point in time. Maybe if Mr. Waters had bought a different house, he would have never fallen in love with the house that was worth more than 3 years in a nursing home. Maybe if the female had a slightly different diet growing up, she would not have developed appendicitis. In this very wide sense of "preventable," almost anything is preventable.

But that is not the concept of preventable that the authors are using by the end of the quote. Instead, they have introduced a new concept of preventable, i.e., some clinical outcome X is preventable only if X is caused by processes that are under the control of clinicians. Policies around handwashing are under the control of clinicians, so clinical outcomes caused by different patterns of handwashing are preventable. But which house Mr. Water bought or what kinds of food the female patient ate as a child are obviously not under control of clinical staff. Any medical complications that arise from these (very distantly!) antecedent conditions are not causes of preventable errors. So, there are two concepts of prevention in play.

The most important observation that we have to offer from our efforts to unpack these three concepts is the observation that, together, these concepts imply a kind of moral prerogative: administrators should try to control the spaces in which patients are treated, in order to ensure that they are only exposed to highly standardized "processes of care," thereby minimizing the risk of preventable injury or death. In practice, this often shows up by creating quality assurance teams who are responsible for designing patient safety metrics and protocols—and these efforts contribute to the further standardization of how care is delivered.

Consequently, it is quite hard to find well-run hospitals, outpatient clinics, and long-term care facilities that do not have a meaningful commitment to the patient safety paradigm. What this involves is putting into practice the three concepts that we extracted from the quote above: care delivery systems should be standardized, the delivery systems themselves are the cause of good or bad outcomes for older persons (i.e., individuals aren't *directly* morally responsible for patient outcomes unless they do not adhere to the standardized processes), and prevention refers only to those actions or outcomes which can be directly tied, causally speaking, to the care delivery systems that are under the control of clinicians. The authors of the report draw the logical conclusion: "standardization and simplification are two fundamental human factors" that are direct causes of safety (Institute of Medicine (US) Committee on Quality of Health Care in America 2000, 156).

8.4 How to Understand "Not Safe at Home"?

We want to connect the association between standardization, simplification, and safety with our early arguments about Maslow, but that will have to wait for just a bit. Here, it is more important to focus on what the forgoing analysis helps us to hear and understand when a clinician says that someone like Mr. Waters is "not safe at home." This utterance probably means something like "Mr. Waters' home is not a place where clinicians are in control (i.e., he does not have systems of care that can be systematized and analyzed for weaknesses). All sorts of things *could happen* to Mr. Waters that *would be preventable*—like his fall! If Mr. Waters came to live in a nursing home rather than staying in his house, we could monitor his care for safety." In other words, assessments that an older person is "not safe at home" can sometimes mean that an older person's home is not a place where the patient safety paradigm operates. It is also an assessment that is made by seeing the older adult in a clinical space (e.g., outpatient clinic, emergency department) and *not* an assessment of how the older adult functions in their home.

But it is obviously absurd to want the paradigm to either apply universally or at least apply in homes and similar private spaces. Why? Homes and similar private spaces are, by definition, places where our unique autonomy can express ourselves. In fact, Mr. Waters' home is almost an inversion of a clinical space organized around older person safety: at home, Mr. Waters is responsible for his actions as an individual, there are not care delivery systems that have been standardized which shape his daily activities and guard him against adverse outcomes, and because of both, there are all sorts of things that could happen to Mr. Waters that, technically, are not preventable errors (even if they would be regarded as preventable errors if they occurred in a clinical setting).

This is not to say that there are no regulations that govern the safety of private residences, for example, certain regulations prevent the sale of lead-based paint or require hardwired smoke alarms. Still, these laws and regulations do not dictate what color paint a homeowner can select for their interior spaces. So, a home should not be thought of as a clinical space or a hospital. When a clinician assesses that an older adult like Mr. Waters is "not safe at home," we invite them and the older adult's families to ask follow-up questions that probe whether this assessment is ultimately grounded in the (usually correct!) perception that the patient safety paradigm does not apply to the older person's home.

8.5 Back to Maslow

The argument that we have developed in this chapter shows that there is a tension between the patient safety paradigm and autonomy. In fact, this tension is easy to see if you have ever stayed overnight in a hospital. Hospitalized individuals almost always must give up—literally sign over, as most hospitals now require patients to sign waivers and terms-of-service agreements upon admission—a tremendous amount of autonomy to receive access to care. But to the extent that a patient is in the hospital only to have their most fundamental capacities restored—remember that the lowest level of Maslow's hierarchy refers to homeostasis—there is a tremendous amount of congruence between a hospital organized according to the patient safety paradigm and an older person's objective ethical needs and interests. Someone in their 30s or 40s may temporarily give up a large amount of their autonomy to have their appendix removed or a fractured bone set back in place and have both operations done without any preventable errors.

But older adults are in a different situation. For many, care is not temporary: it is a permanent feature for the rest of their life. And while it may be reasonable from time to time for older adults to give up autonomy for access to medical care, our view is that these should be exceptional circumstances, rather than the default operating principle when caring for adults. Another way of putting the point we are making in this chapter, then, is that standardization and simplification cause us to focus only on the lowest level of anyone's pyramid of needs. A temporary focus on the lowest level may be rational for most people, but that is a very different idea that, as soon as someone needs permanent care, it is appropriate to try to simplify and standardize most of their life. Please look back at the illustration of Mr. Kane's pyramid from Chap. 1; we like this picture because it is *not* a picture of a life that has been standardized and simplified. Mr. Kane's life, like anyone's life, is a tangled mess. Our argument is that too much of a focus on safety—and not enough of a focus on the elements higher up in the pyramid—deprives older persons of any number of ethically important things, like boysenberry pie or access to their own home. Rather than resorting to simplification (often over simplification that results from trying to standardize environments), we believe it is important to render the complexity accessible so that we can build our care processes and practices around the unique needs, values, and preferences of each older adult.

8.6 Death Is Not a Preventable Error in Older Adults

The final observation we want to offer you in this chapter is, in a sentence, death is not a preventable error in older adults. The prevalence of death in humans is 100%. And while some adverse events are preventable, the risk that something bad is going to happen to an older adult rises with age, with frailty, with dementia, and with decrements in functional and cognitive capacity. It is logically impossible to make safety—if safety means preventing any of these outcomes—the most important principle in the care of older adults. This gives Terri's favorite question—"What were you hoping would happen?"—a new meaning. Before, we suggested that it was not reasonable to think that a person who, upon moving into a nursing home, would become a totally new person. Patterns in the person's life would continue pretty much as they always have. The same applies here with regard to safety. Adverse events will occur in the lives of all individuals, no matter where they live or how they are cared for. The cold, hard truth is that, despite all our systems and standards and processes, we simply cannot prevent all the bad things that could happen to an older adult (to anyone, actually). So, when someone says "Mr. Waters is no longer safe at home," it is important to not be misled into thinking "Well, Mr. Waters would be safe in the nursing home!". We can try to construct a metaphorical safety net around older adults, but the distance between the net and the older adult must be tailored to each individual situation.

8.7 The Prevalence of Autonomy and Value

We do not need only to focus on negative outcomes when thinking about prevalence rates for older adults. Positive things have a certain prevalence rate, too. Mr. Kane from Chap. 1 and Mr. Waters here both get value from important features of their lives: boysenberry pie and living in a cherished home. Too much of a focus on safety can cause us to ignore the ways in which decisions about an older adult's care can dramatically alter the frequency that "good things" (pie! Waking up in one's home!) occur in people's lives. Attending to the prevalence of good things matters as much, if not more, as older persons age, because these rates are at risk of declining, roughly in proportion to the rise in risk of adverse events and resulting efforts to promote safety.

So, another helpful thing to keep in mind when you hear someone say something like "She is not safe at home" or "Your mother will be much safer if she moves to the nursing home!" is to think about how moving into a nursing will change the prevalence rate of experiences of value or expressions of autonomy. We caution specifically about accepting a change that trades away nearly all expressions of autonomy of experiences of value for what might, realistically, be a small change in the underlying base rate occurence of adverse events. As Mr. Waters put it especially vividly, sometimes, these kinds of trades don't make any sense.

Discussion and Reflection Questions

1. Just like past chapters, this chapter highlights the tension between a provider's concern for safety and an older adult's desire for autonomy or how they define quality of life. How can future healthcare professionals navigate situations like

Mr. Waters', where an older person's preference for independence seemingly conflicts with perceived safety risks?

2. The chapter discusses how the "patient safety paradigm" emphasizes standardized care and system-level error prevention. How might this paradigm inadvertently limit the quality of life or autonomy for older adults in their own homes?
3. We know that certain adverse events, like falls or even death, are highly prevalent in older populations and not always preventable errors. How can understanding the notion that not all negative outcomes are preventable influence prioritizing safety for older adults?

References

Bates DW, Singh H (2018) Two decades since to err is human: an assessment of progress and emerging priorities in older person safety. Health Aff (Project Hope) 37(11):1736–1743

Institute of Medicine (US) Committee on Quality of Health Care in America (2000) To err is human: building a safer health system. National Academies Press (US), Washington, DC

Sharp HM, Bryant KN (2003) Ethical issues in dysphagia: when older persons refuse assessment or treatment. Semin Speech Lang 24(4):285–299

Yardley L, Donovan-Hall M, Francis K, Todd C (2006) Older people's views of advice about falls prevention: a qualitative study. Health Educ Res 21(4):508–517

9 Our Suggestions for Dealing with Impossible Choices

9.1 Wrapping Up

As you can see, this chapter does not begin with a case. That is because we are near the end of sharing our ideas about how to think about caring for older adults. Since we've covered a lot of ground, we want to start wrapping up by summarizing the advice that we are offering.

It is actually a bit much to call it advice: an impossible choice is a choice that you must make and about which you will probably never have certainty as to whether you made the right or the wrong choice. These choices are extremely stressful. Life forces impossible choices on us, and it is usually exhausting to try to reason your way through them, because reason just keeps looking for a solution or the "right" solution and keeps coming up empty. The only way to deal with an impossible choice is to go through it. But that means any recommendations that we offer you really have the characteristics of a mixture of empathy and hope: we've shared some ideas with you, and we hope that these ideas help you feel a little less isolated and overwhelmed by any impossible choices that you are facing. Maybe some of the ideas can help identify ways of reducing the burdens of the situation a little bit or at least provide some context and perspective as to why things are so stuck. But, sadly, we cannot offer you a recipe, a strategy, or an algorithm for dealing with impossible choices in the case of older adults. Believe us, if we thought we could, we would!

Instead, what we have to offer is a "bag" of suggestions, big and small, that can be that source of context of perspective. We call this a "bag" of suggestions because the ideas can all be held together, but none of the ideas is more important than the other. You can take the suggestions out and try them in whichever order you want; they don't form some kind of overarching scientific or logical structure. They are ideas that we have collected from our combined clinical experience and scientific training and research—so they are suggestions that we carry with us. In a way, this book is an attempt to share our bag of ideas for thinking through the care of the elderly with you. Maybe you will carry some of these ideas that work best for you

T. A. Harvath, M. Fedyk, *What If Maslow Was Wrong?*,
https://doi.org/10.1007/978-3-032-14249-8_9

along your journey in caring for the elderly. And we certainly hope that you add to the bag! It has room for many more suggestions!

So, here then is a quick summary of nine suggestions that capture much of what we've tried to convey so far:

1. *Impossible Choices Are Normal*

   Caring for older adults sooner or later gives rise to impossible choices. These are choices that cannot be avoided: we must pick either A or B or "none of the above" sooner or later. But the nature of the choice is that we will never be certain that we made the right choice, and before making the choice, it is usually impossible to have sufficient evidence that the choice being made is right. Consequently, when faced with an impossible choice, it is important to have compassion for yourself and everyone else involved in the situation—and it is equally important to try, if possible, to avoid exhausting yourself by looking for either more evidence ("if only I can figure this out, then I'll know what to do!") or persistently avoiding making a choice ("I can keep going like this forever!"). Impossible choices are especially exhausting, and a sequence of impossible choices can wear down even the strongest clinicians, families, friendships, or marriages.
2. *What If Maslow Were Wrong? (Balancing* Versus *Maximizing)*

   We have titled this book *What If Maslow Was Wrong?* because we want to get your attention and to show that there are alternative ways of thinking about safety in the care of older adults beyond "maximizing safety" or "putting safety first." Maslow's hierarchy of needs is one of the most influential scientific ideas that shapes clinician thinking about safety, so by understanding that Maslow himself did not think that safety should be maximized but also that the higher needs associated with self-actualization have "organic unity" in a person's life means that we can take a "balancing" attitude toward safety: it is one of several things to try to conserve or maintain in life. As a result, if you are caring for an older adult, "tall and skinny" pyramids are to be preferred to "wide and flat" pyramids.
3. *The Word "Safety" Means Different Things: Normal Accidents Are Predictable*

   The word "safety" has several standard meanings when used in the context of the care of older adults: usually, error reduction and risk mitigation. What is important to understand, however, is that normal accidents—breakdowns in the social systems that prevent error or mitigate risk—are a predictable by-product of trying to build safe clinics, nursing homes, assisted living facilities, and so on. No safety-generating social system is risk-free or immune to errors. Because absolute safety is not possible, what else needs to be considered when making decisions on behalf of older adults?
4. *Weighing Costs and Benefits Can Sometimes Help Make Decisions*

   One of the simplest alternatives to making choices that are designed to maximize safety is to make decisions according to cost-benefit analysis. Do your best to estimate the value of different pros and cons associated with different choices, add up the values assigned to the various pros and cons, and go with the choice that seems like it will generate the most value for everyone involved.

5. *Use the Mental Model of A Wobbly Three-Legged Stool to Think About Balancing Autonomy, Quality of Life, and Safety*

   If cost-benefit thinking is too complex, using a "three-legged stool" model is a simpler alternative that often leads to the same results. The mental model helps you creatively seek out ways to balance safety, autonomy, and quality of life—it prevents you from focusing too much on just one of any of the three "legs." We have explained why focusing on all three legs can be hard for most providers to do in practice. But by keeping in mind that the stool is already wobbling and that the goal isn't to make it perfectly stable but instead just make sure that it doesn't tip over, both patients and providers will see the utility (we hope).
6. *A "Safety-First" Strategy Can Easily Backfire*

   An important caution against trying to solve impossible choices by pursuing safety is that, very often, this can backfire.
7. *Autonomy Isn't Independence, and It Doesn't Disappear as Capacities Dimmish*

   Don't conflate independence and autonomy, and there are various ways—such as looking for long-standing patterns in a person's life that can be continued despite diminishing capacities—of preserving a person's autonomy. Again, we should prefer tall and skinny pyramids of needs to short and flat pyramids.
8. *Being a Kantian Sometimes Helps, but Being An Ethical Pragmatist Is Always an Option Too*

   You can be a Kantian about impossible choices if you try to find ways forward that promote a patient's autonomy as much as possible—by asking which choices express "ends for their own sake" or which "retain the humanity" of a patient with dimentia. Given how much emphasis nursing homes and long-term care facilities and hospitals place on safety, ensure that attention is also paid to autonomy and quality of life, even for—especially for—older adults with decreased decisional capacity. But at the same time, concepts like "ends" and "retained humanity" can be hard to reconcile with the complexity of clinical environment. When this happens, the ethical pragmatist's rule "Without making things worse, try to discover how to make things better" can be a useful for discovering how to make marginal ethical improvements.
9. *The Prevalence of Accidents or Irreversible Illness Increases with Age*

   This simple truth is perhaps the most important rule of all: we should not try to find solutions to care of older adults that somehow defy the consequences of these generalizations. Avoid thinking that increasing the amount of safety in a person's life is a way of compensating for the increase in the amount of risk. This is both a mathematical and a sociological mistake. But it becomes a moral mistake when maximizing safety becomes a reason to strip a person of their autonomy. No one is going to live forever, but everyone has the possibility of living nearly all their life in a way that is mostly congruent with their deepest values.

9.2 How to Use the Suggestions

We stress that the suggestions are *only* suggestions. Each of them can be helpful in navigating decisions about care for older adults (and perhaps even for younger adults, but we digress); each help provides some important context for those decisions. But none of the ideas should be taken as a fixed rule or general principle for decision-making. We have shared with you cases that exemplify our suggestions—but we have both encountered other cases where following any of the suggestions would be completely the wrong thing to do. This means that, ultimately, we encourage you to, first, mix and match the ideas and, second, when the ideas seem to run out of value for you, try to invent your own. Here, the goal shouldn't be to create ethical certainty—to find the optimal, or right, or best choice. Instead, the goal should be just to build more context for the choices, impossible or otherwise, that you are facing.

9.3 The Most Important Suggestion of All: Don't Forget to Be Kind to the Little Person

Why? Well, as we've said, impossible choices exhaust those who face them. It is all too easy to believe that just a bit more reasoning or research will uncover a new option about how to proceed; a bit more cognitive effort will uncover some more justified, more certain, more evidence-based choice. Eventually, impossible choices wear a person down, because "do more thinking" or "just apply a different combination of rules" is unfortunately not a strategy for solving impossible choices. Sooner or later, the choice just must be made.

Because of this, we want to conclude this book with two stories that distill a different kind of ethical wisdom than is expressed in the ten suggestions above. Both of these stories are from Terri's life; both are stories about what it is like to face an impossible choice, move through making the impossible choice, and then dealing with the emotional consequences of having made an impossible choice. The second of these stories comes from Terri's life right now, and it walks us through the whole process of facing an impossible choice involving the care of Terri's elderly mother; it shows you how Terri worked through the ethical challenges of a deeply personal impossible choice. Since it is the longer story, it takes up the postscript that follows this concluding chapter.

The first of these stories is just below, coming in the form of a letter (edited to preserve anonymity) that Terri wrote to Phillip, who had been appointed durable power of attorney on behalf of George, who was near death due to cancer. George was one of both Terri' and Phillip's closest friends. Phillip had spent several months arguing with George's sister about all sorts of different impossible choices that had to be made for George. The important thing about this letter is that it was George who first taught Terri how to write such letters. George was a pediatric nurse, and so would, at times, talk to the "little people" inside of all adults whenever he felt that the rational self was getting in the way or taking up too much space. Terri wrote this letter to Phillip just as his exhaustion from dealing with impossible choices about George's care was pushing him past his mental limits.

Dear Little Person,

I know Phillip usually reads emails from me, but I'd like to talk with you, his little person, for a minute.

You see, Philip is a very responsible adult, and he is really good at that, but sometimes he does that a little bit too well and makes the mistake that a lot of adults make in thinking that there are singular right answers to some of life's most difficult issues.

So, I'd like to ask you to help Philip understand the difference between making the right decision and making a decision the right way, because even though you are little, you know something about this. You see, Philip's best friend, George, asked Philip to do something really hard—George asked Philip to make decisions on Philip's behalf in case he couldn't do that himself. And that is a really big responsibility. George thought about asking other people to do that, but he realized that Philip was the best one for this hard job because he would take this responsibility seriously; George was counting on Philip's tendency to be a very responsible adult. I think George understood that Philip would work really hard to make the decision that George would make for himself if he had the capacity to do so. He didn't want someone who would make a decision because they thought it was in George's best interest, usurping his autonomy. The only problem is that while George was clear about what he wanted in the beginning, he got scared and confused, and this made it hard to know what he wanted later on when he was really, really sick. The part I need your help with is to help Philip understand that the decision per se *was not the most important part of what George asked Philip to do. The most important part was the way Philip went about making the decision, the struggle to try to make the decision that George had hoped to make for himself, the decision George tried to make in advance through the addendum to his advance directives. I think George knew that when he was at his most vulnerable, Philip would wrestle with the decision instead of thinking he just knew what was best for George. What I hope for Philip's big person is that he can see that he gave George the ultimate gift, which was assuring George that the trust he placed in Philip was the right decision.*

When you and Philip read this, he might try to put up all sorts of logical arguments. Please help him see that this is not a matter that is best understood through logic. This is one of those issues that must be understood through the heart. So please tell Philip's head to politely take a hike and listen to his heart, to you on this issue.

With love,

Terri's little person, doing her level best to channel George

Terri's letter lets us show you one of the most important lessons for nurses, doctors, students, families, friends, wives, and husbands—all the people who provide care for older adults. Nothing matters more—not autonomy, not quality of life, not safety, and certainly not any of the ten suggestions we offered above—than being kind and loving toward yourself as you wrestle with impossible choices. Rather than trying to maximize or prioritize safety, we suggest that you try never to forget that there is a "little person" inside all of us—someone who needs love and kindness much more than they need the logically correct answers to truly impossible problem.

My Own Caregiving Experiences

Over the years it took to conceive and write this book, I (Terri) have had some personal experiences with caring for older family members. My parents lived in a single-story ranch-style home that had three bedrooms and a bathroom on the main floor and a bathroom with a shower in the basement. They had lived in that house since 1970, and no one had ever used the shower on the main floor. In 2008, my dad had hip replacement surgery. I stayed with my parents for a week following his discharge from inpatient rehabilitation. When my dad wanted to take a shower, I suggested that it would be easier to use the one on the main floor. They both said no to that. You see, there was a window in that bathroom that was within the tub/shower enclosure, and they did not want that window to get wet and ruin the wooden sill. I suggested we could cover the window with plastic to protect it, but they were adamant that the only place to shower was in the basement. So, to get to the basement, my mom went down the narrow stairs first and my dad followed her, one step at a time. As I watched this, I could only imagine how dangerous this was for both of them. One misstep and they would both end up in a heap at the bottom of the stairs, with broken necks—because that is how the mind works when the safety of one's parents is involved.

I watched this scene unfold but had the presence of mind not to interfere (not because I was observing in order to gather clinical data but because I was afraid if I said anything they would lose their focus and the fall would be my fault!). The next time my dad wanted a shower, I raised some objections, but they again insisted this was safe. To prove it to me, they had me go first down the stairs with my dad trailing (I suppose so that I could go down in a blaze of glory and break my neck when he stumbled—again the active imagination of a concerned daughter at work).

After this shower, I sat with them to discuss my concerns about this arrangement. I said I didn't think it was safe. They both assured me that they were careful and held on to the railing as they descended. I said it would be easy for us to remodel their current bathroom to make the shower easy to get in, to protect the window, and we could even get the laundry on the main floor, up from the basement. Afterall, one brother is a pipe fitter and could do the plumbing, and my other brothers who lived locally could help with the carpentry work. My parents were adamant that they did not want the laundry on the main floor: What if the washing machine broke, they

T. A. Harvath, M. Fedyk, *What If Maslow Was Wrong?*,
https://doi.org/10.1007/978-3-032-14249-8

would get water damage throughout the first floor and damage the hardwood floors. So, I said, "Would you rather risk falling down the steps and breaking your necks and lying on the basement floor in agony until someone found you than move the shower and laundry to the main floor?" The answer was an unequivocable yes! Well, I decided I had done my best, and this is what they wanted, so I decided to let it be.

About a week later, my oldest brother was visiting and witnessed the "decent-of-the-basement-stairs-in-order-to-shower" process. He called me and we had the following conversation:

Brother: "Do you know what they are doing when dad needs a shower?"
Me: "Yes, I witnessed that just the week before."
Brother: "They are both going to fall down those steps and break their necks!" (Apparently concerned brothers share an active imagination with their concerned sister.)
Me: "Yes, I told them the same thing. They said they would rather fall down the steps, break their necks, and lay there in agony than move the shower and laundry upstairs."
Brother: "Oh, well, I guess if they know the risks, it is their decision."

And while I had secretly hoped that my brother would not accept their decision and we could gang up on them and convince them to move the shower and laundry to the main floor, I knew he was right. And so, we never again suggested they move the shower and laundry to the main floor. And they never did fall down those steps. And they never did break their necks and lay in agony on the basement floor. And the hardwood floors and the windowsill were saved from water damage. And I learned how hard it is to realize that there are limits to our ability to protect the ones we love from all the dangers we can imagine may befall them. And I learned (maybe) how to accept risk to protect my parents' autonomy and their quality of life.

Fast forward a few years and my mom had moved into a two-bedroom duplex following the death of my dad. She was a few years older and had bad knees and struggled to get up and down stairs. Thankfully, the shower for the duplex was on the main floor; unfortunately, the laundry was in the basement. My sisters and I offered to do her laundry for her, but she insisted she could do it. My mother is a very independent woman and takes pride in being able to manage on her own. She did not want to cede responsibility for laundry to her daughters. We once again had the conversation about her falling down the basement steps, breaking her neck, and laying in agony until she was found. She insisted that her independence was worth the risk. And besides, she told me she was careful. So, I advocated for her to be able to do her laundry as she wished. And she never fell down those steps. And she never broke her neck and laid in agony until someone found her. And once again, I had the uneasy task of accepting risk on behalf of her autonomy.

After my mother (voluntarily) gave up her car and driving, one of the duties assigned to me was to take my mom on her "big" grocery shopping trips. We made these trips five to six times each year during nice weather. These trips included a stop at a discount variety store where she stocked up on toilet paper, tissue, and cleaning supplies as well as candy and snacks that she wanted to have on hand for when anyone visited. Then, we would go to a big box grocery store where she would stock up on canned goods, catsup (she would get about 20 bottles of catsup each year!), and any meat that was on sale that she would put in her freezer. She would spend between $400 and $500 on these excursions. She wanted to be stocked up so that she wouldn't need much during the winter months when it was icy.

To take my mom shopping meant that I would pick her up, stand by while she got down the steps to her duplex, and give her my arm so we could walk slowly to my car. Then, we would park, and I would give her my arm so we could walk slowly to the store. As soon as she got behind a grocery cart, that woman would canvas the store with purpose and a strong quick stride. She would send me off to find an item, and once the item was in hand, I had to search multiple aisles to find her as she kept a brisk pace (in contrast to her slow and cautious gait without the support of the grocery cart).

One of my sisters had gotten my mom a really nice purple four-wheeled walker at a thrift store for $30. It had brakes and a seat. She refused to use it, saying she didn't need it. In an aside, I told my sister she should have gotten mom a grocery cart instead. I guess there is less stigma to using a grocery cart than a walker as we age! Again, a lesson in how to respect and preserve her autonomy!

A few months ago, my mom got a sinus infection. It triggered an exacerbation of her congestive heart failure and her COPD. She stopped eating and drinking because it was too much of a burden. Then one day, my sister called, saying mom had fallen and couldn't get up. Mom was taken to the ER where they ordered some antibiotics and called in case management. We arranged for her to go on hospice, per her request, so that she wouldn't have to go to the hospital anymore. She asked to see a priest and said she was ready to die. She moved in with one of my sisters for a few weeks and started to get better; then, she moved in with me.

Her first week here was a little rough for me. She commented on all the jars of condiments in my refrigerator wondering who needs all that other stuff (all she has is catsup). She suggested that I could arrange my furniture differently to make more space in the living room. The food I cooked was "interesting." Each of these comments caused me silent irritation.

By the second week, I had learned her morning routine and could anticipate her needs. She awakened at six to pray, telling me "I say prayers for a lot of people, and they are not going to get said on their own! I have to get going on that." My sister called at 7:50 am every morning to check on her (a holdover from the pandemic when my siblings and I had a schedule for calling her each day). Then, she would get washed up and dressed so that at 9:15 am she could listen to mass on her phone (if she could get it—never a sure thing). While she listened to mass, I made her toast and coffee, got her a fresh glass of water and some V8. I found that I enjoyed doing these things for her, and she seemed pleased that I had learned what she liked. I settled into the caregiving role, realizing that she was gaining strength, and this could be a long-term arrangement instead of a short-term hospice gig.

My mom has always liked playing cards, so we started playing Casino, a card game she had played with my dad to see who had to do the dishes after they became empty nesters. We'd play a couple games after lunch and a couple after dinner. At first, we were just playing and tracking who was winning. Initially, I did it just to humor her, to give her something to break up what I believed was the monotony of her day. Then, I started tallying who had won the most games and who had skunked the other person, and she was ahead(!) (my mom will be the first to tell you that we are all competitive, most especially her).

At one point, we decided to play for a dime each game. I found I started to look forward to our games and the friendly competition. Sometimes, she would mix up the cards that would be dealt with the discards, and we'd have to scrap that hand. Sometimes, she would miss some obvious plays, perhaps because of a little memory problem or if she was tired. At first, I would point these mistakes out to her and try to let her have the replay. She would have none of that. If she missed it (regardless of the cause), she missed it. At first, I felt bad, like I was cheating if her missed play threw the hand my way. Then, I realized that despite those lapses she was winning a fair number of times. Then, I felt bad that I couldn't beat my 93-year-old mother at cards, even when she was missing plays!

Gradually, my mom started to get stronger. Those of us who work in gerontology know that it is very difficult to predict who will die and when. The antibiotics that had been ordered in the ER seemed to have helped. The stronger she got, the more she started meddling in my kitchen! At first, it was kind of sweet. I had always been her helper in the kitchen growing up, and being in the kitchen with her again brought up fond memories for both of us. But then she wanted to have input into meal planning and making suggestions on what I was cooking and how. I could feel some irritation return. I then realized that she was now treading on "my" sense of autonomy (after all, I had been cooking for myself for years without her help), and I had to chuckle to myself. So, this is what that feels like!

After a few weeks, she started to say that she wanted to get her own assisted living (AL) apartment. Despite my telling her she could stay with me, she was clear that she preferred to live on her own (if I'm honest, I was relieved). So, we started looking for an AL apartment. We found one that seemed to have what she liked, but when she heard the cost, she balked. She thought perhaps she could just live in independent living to save money. Six weeks after moving in with me, we moved her into her own one-bedroom apartment in a senior living complex.

Despite her long history of a poor sense of direction, she has learned how to get around her new apartment complex. She is able to find the chapel where she can attend mass three times each week and rosary every day. She manages to dump her trash bag down the chute despite the heavy door that needs to be held open. She has laundry facilities in her unit and is happy to be able to do her own laundry again (and my sisters and I are relieved that she is not going upstairs and downstairs for laundry!). She has started using her purple four-wheeled walker to get around outside the apartment because of the distance, something she was never willing to do before insisting she didn't need it.

A couple months ago, she fell and fractured her pelvis in two places. She was hospitalized but didn't require surgery. She was transferred to a transitional care unit to have physical and occupational therapy. It turns out you heal pelvic fractures by bearing weight—something that was very painful for my mom. Still, she was determined to return to independent living, and after two and a half weeks, she went back to her apartment! Her desire for independence remains strong!

This journey of caregiving is not over. My mother seems to have more gas in her tank than we gave her credit for. It has been humbling, rewarding, irksome, wonderful, and surprising to experience caregiving and to live with the risks to someone I love. It reminds me of conversations I had with my daughter as she was growing up when I realized her desire for independence and autonomy would always outpace my comfort with it!

I still live with some uneasiness about her living independently. She turns the sound on her phone off when she goes to mass or rosary and often forgets to turn it back on. When one of my siblings calls to check on her and can't reach her, they will call my sister and me to check on her. I get a sinking feeling as we drive toward her apartment, wondering if we are going to find her on the floor, wondering whether she may have died (peacefully, I always hope). So far, I have not yet made it all the way to her apartment (30 minutes away) before she calls to apologize for having forgotten to turn her ringer back on.

But it is a reminder of the discomfort I feel in "allowing" (as if it is my decision) her to live independently. I think about how I will feel if something "bad" happens to her. Will my siblings blame me? Will I blame myself for not insisting on the assisted living facility where I could at least call someone to go check on her. Was I wrong in advocating for her independence and autonomy? I cannot know the answer to any of these questions—they are impossible choices. However, I feel like holding me discomfort with her autonomy is the right thing to do. My mom has thanked me repeatedly for "allowing" her to do her own laundry while in the duplex. It is a reminder to me that there are worse things than breaking a hip and dying for some people. Losing independence, losing autonomy is a form of suffering that is real and significant. And while I am not able to protect my mother from all the bad things that could happen to her, I am able to try to protect her autonomy. In doing so, I believe I am also protecting her quality of life.

Advance Directives: Additional Instructions[1]

This document serves as additional instructions as to my wishes and preferences regarding healthcare treatment decisions in the event I cannot consent or refuse treatment because of diminished decisional capacity.

As a nurse, I have seen many families struggle with surrogate decision-making because the exact situation they are facing does not match the healthcare directives signed by their relative. Therefore, I can only hope that this document provides some additional guidance to those who may be required to make difficult decisions on my behalf.

At this point in my life, what is important and meaningful for me is to be able to engage fully in my relationships with others. By this, I mean that it is important for me to be able to laugh, cry, and debate with others in ways that engage my full intellectual and emotional capacities. It is important to me to be able to converse with others, to listen and hear what others have to say, to participate in conversations in deep, meaningful, and substantial ways. To be clear, I don't consider things like eye blinking or hand squeezing to constitute meaningful engagement in conversation (and I fully respect that for others this can be part of a meaningful life). If, at some point in the future, I am not able to engage in meaningful interactions with others, I don't believe I will have the quality of life that is valuable to me. For me, quality of life is much more important than quantity of life. If I have an illness, accident, or injury that prevents me from engaging in human relationships in meaningful ways, I would *not* want to be sustained on life support or through artificial foods and fluids (e.g., tube feedings, intravenous fluids, etc.). If it is unclear whether I will recover, I am willing to have a brief (i.e., few weeks, not months) course of treatment to see if recovery to a meaningful level is possible. But I would want that decision reviewed after 4–6 weeks, and if I have not made substantial gains (i.e., regained my capacity to engage meaningfully with others), please remove those life-sustaining

[1] Please feel free to use any or all of this document to craft your own individual advanced directives.

T. A. Harvath, M. Fedyk, *What If Maslow Was Wrong?*,
https://doi.org/10.1007/978-3-032-14249-8

interventions, and let me go. If there are doubts as to my recovery, I would rather have my surrogates err on the side of letting me go rather than maintaining me in a state of ambiguity or, worse, a state where I am incapable of interaction or, worst of all, a state where I know what is going on around me but am unable to communicate with others. If you are unable to withdraw a life-sustaining treatment, then please do not start it.

I also recognize that if I am in such a situation, there may be individuals who would find it difficult to let me go. They may hope that I'll be able to recover. To them, I would say please understand that I believe that my physical presence may offer short-term comfort and be a place where hope might reside. However, I also believe that it would become burdensome and the memories of me being in that suspended state of living would become difficult to live with. Even if you disagree with my assessment of what constitutes quality of life, please respect my wishes.

So, if I am having pain or severe shortness of breath, I would want medications that might ease my suffering, even if it hastens my death by depressing my respirations or otherwise causes adverse consequences. If you are uncertain, assume I'm suffering and keep me comfortable. I would also prefer not to be treated with antibiotics if doing so merely prolongs my living in a state that does not represent quality of life.

As someone who has worked with older adults and families with dementia, I also recognize the possibility of being in a situation where I have significant cognitive impairment but am physically in fairly good shape. I have seen any number of individuals who no longer recognize their families but seem to have pleasant days as they move among the staff of a congregate living situation. On the surface, that can look like a reasonable quality of life. For me, however, I go back to wanting to be able to engage in meaningful conversations with people whom I know, recognize, and love. So even if I am the "belle of the nursing home" (I can only hope that I would be ☺), please know that still doesn't reach the standard of quality of life that I value. So, if I'm in that situation and I get pneumonia or some other life-threatening illness, please do not treat me to prolong my life. Only treat me for comfort, even if it hastens my death.

Also, if I have dementia and you find that I am irritable or aggressive, please recognize that it is not my baseline personality (at least I don't think it is) and that it may mean that something is wrong (e.g., pain, hunger, constipation, etc.) that needs to be addressed. Please try to address those needs. If, however, you cannot find anything that prevents me from hitting other people or being mean or nasty, then please medicate me, even if it means sedating me and might hasten my death. I would rather be "snowed" than aggressive toward others.

I also recognize that during the end-of-life process, I might develop delirium. If asked whether I would want life-saving or life-sustaining measures, I might respond that I want to be kept alive. DON'T LISTEN TO THAT PERSON! I would ask that you recognize this statement, that I am creating now (and one that I review periodically to ensure it still expresses my sincere advance directives), as the truest expression of my wishes.

I would also like to offer a word about my care in a long-term care setting (e.g., assisted living, memory care, nursing home, etc.). I have never been a morning person. And although my work situation has often required me to get up early, it is *not* something that I want to have in retirement or in long-term care. My preference is that I be allowed to sleep until I awaken of my own accord, even if it means missing breakfast. Then, I would love to lie in bed with a cup of good coffee (black) reading the newspaper (preferably the *New York Times*) until such time I am ready to get out of bed. If I have dementia, I might still want the paper, even if it is the same paper every morning simply because it is a ritual I enjoy.

I hope that these statements help with the difficult decisions that surrogates are sometimes called upon to make.

GPSR Compliance

The European Union's (EU) General Product Safety Regulation (GPSR) is a set of rules that requires consumer products to be safe and our obligations to ensure this.

If you have any concerns about our products, you can contact us on ProductSafety@springernature.com

In case Publisher is established outside the EU, the EU authorized representative is:

Springer Nature Customer Service Center GmbH
Europaplatz 3
69115 Heidelberg, Germany

Batch number: 10370712

Printed by Printforce, the Netherlands